Cannabis for Seniors

Beverly A. Potter, Ph.D.

"Docpotter"

RONIN

Berkeley, California

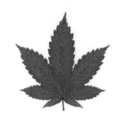

Important Notice:

Information in this book is provided under the First Amendment of the Constitution and is not medical advice. Readers should discuss issues raised in this book with their personal physician and follow their physician's advice regarding it. Readers should also consult an attorney as to the legal status of cannabis in their state and city.

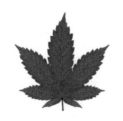

Cannabis for Seniors

Beverly A. Potter, Ph.D.

"Docpotter"

Cannabis for Seniors

Copyright 2017 by Beverly A. Potter
ISBN: 978-1-57951-242-2 Pbook
ISBN: 9781579512439 Ebook

Published by

Ronin Publishing, Inc.
PO Box 3436
Oakland, CA 94609
www.roninpub.com

Production:
  Manuscript creaton: Beverly A. Potter.
  Cover Design: Brian Groppe.
  Book Design: Beverly A. Potter.
  Content Creation: Abby Hauck/CannabisContent.com
  Photos: Fotolia

Library of Congress Card Number: 2017902698
Manufactured in the United States by Lightning Source.
Distributed to the book trade by PGW/Ingram.

Acknowledgements

Thank you, Dear Reader, for picking up this book. May you find comfort and inspiration in the information shared here in.

A special thanks to Abby Hauck and her team, and to Mark Schapiro for your invaluable contributions to *Cannabis for Seniors*.

—Docpotter

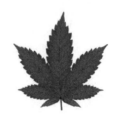

You can't stop getting older, but you don't have to get old.

Table of Contents

1. Why Cannabis for Seniors?............ 9
2. The Endocannabinoid System 14
3. Cannabis Myths 25
4. Routes into the Bloodstream 32
5. How to Use Cannabis 41
6. Therapeutic Strains 51
7. Tailor Your Therapeutics 58
8. Senior Opioid Epidemic 66
9. Reducing Opioid Dependency 73
10. Cannabis and Depression 80
11. Cannabis and Anxiety 90
12. Managing Pain 100
13. Mind/Body Pain Control 110
14. Neuroprotection 120
15. Cannabis and Chemo 131
16. A Good Night's Sleep 137
17. Quelling Discomforts 146
18. Cannabis Promotes Socializing 153
19. Healing Laughter 160
20. Cannabis Topicals 169
21. Cooking with Cannabis 174
22. DIY Cannabis Medicines 185
Bibliography 297
Author Bio 203
Ronin Books for Independent Minds 205

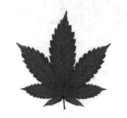

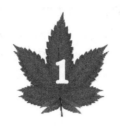

Why Cannabis for Seniors?

Baby boomers are turning 65 to become "Seniors" at an incredible rate of 10,000 each day. The percent of Americans aged 65 or older will grow to 18 percent by 2030 and it is projected that the senior citizens population will balloon to 89 million by 2050. If you've made it to 65, the Centers for Disease Control and Prevention (CDC) predicts that you will live another 19.3 years.

Baby boomers, born between 1946 and 1964, now becoming "Senior Boomers," will dramatically change the business and lifestyle landscape. Senior boomers are predicted to stay in the workforce longer than their parents did, both because

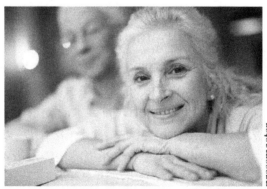

-pressmaster

Senior Boomers will change the landscape of Aging.

they need the money and they're not ready to leave behind fulfilling careers. When they finally do retire, their need for health care and assisted living is predicted to alter what retirement living arrangements look like for generations to come.

Special Issues

Seniors have special issues, the most prominent of which is simple aging—the body wears out. Seniors have all kinds of aches like arthritis, stiff backs, knees, and hips, and muscle spasms. As it turns out cannabis is particularly soothing to muscles and ligaments.

Doctors readily prescribe strong addictive narcotics to seniors to ease these pains and do little monitoring of use, making it easy for seniors to slide into dependency without realizing it. It is not uncommon for seniors to be taking 8 to 10 pills, even more daily. Some report taking 20 pills a day!

It is easy for seniors become isolated. Their spouse may have died and their kids grown. They may be retired and no longer going to a work place every day to interact with co-workers. It is harder to meet new people as a senior. Just getting out and going places by oneself can be a chore; as compared to when back in college when you just stepped out the door in the dorm

to fall in with
other kids go-
ing somewhere.
Seniors are not
likely to go to
a hang out bar,
especially alone.
With isolation
comes feeling
lonely and help-

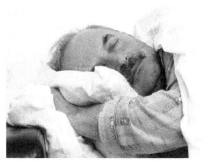

Cannabis promtes restful sleep.

-Sandor Kacso

less to be able to change it can lead to anxiety and
worrying about one's situation and health and
future.

Another frequent issue is getting a good night
sleep. Having difficulty sleeping well seems to
come with aging. Here, again doctors tend to over
prescribe sleeping meds, which when used night-
ly can lead to dependency.

Cannabis has properties and benefits that seniors can draw upon for aid in these issues and to
reduce the amount of strong narcotics and substitute the more benign cannabis therapeutics.

Learning to Use Cannabis

Seniors have had varying degrees of experience
with cannabis. Many are regular users. Others
had a few experiences in college or have been at
parties where joints were passed around that they
may have tried. Others have not had direct expe-

rience, but almost all seniors have seen movies or read books wherein marijuana—pot—was used and enjoyed.

You may have heard that you "must learn to get high". Or heard someone say something like, "I tried it a few times and nothing happened." Sociologist Howard Becker's research shows that when we ingest a drug we have to be "taught" to recognize the effects. For marijuana, the effects usually include heightened senses, food cravings, and sometimes feelings of anxiety, that could progress to paranoia. The first few times we may ignore the effects or get frightened by them—as part of "learning" to use marijuana.

Drinking alcohol is common in our world. But we're not born knowing how to "drink". We've all experienced drinking too much and getting the "whirlies" or stumbling around, even passing out. In these early experiences we learned the feelings and effects of alcohol—what to expect and how to handle it. For some, such early "training" is the first step in becoming a wine connoisseur, which is a very refined "taste".

Learning to Use Cannabis Therapeutics

Learning to use cannabis therapeutically begins with you—an individual, a unique human. It is important to notice how you feel *before* using cannabis—as a baseline for comparison to how you feel *after* employing a particular "therapeutic" use. The emphasis in this book is on cannabis as a therapeutic rather than cannabis as a "medicine". Synonyms of therapeutic include healing, curative, remedial, medicinal, restorative, salubrious, health-giving, tonic, reparative, corrective, beneficial, good, salutary.

When speaking of cannabis many often make a distinction between "recreational" and "medical" cannabis. That is a false distinction. Recreational = re-creational, which is therapeutic. Having fun is beneficial *and* therapeutic. While "passing a joint" is considered recreational, conviviality and laughing with friends is therapeutic.

Synonyms of Therapeutic include *healing, curative, remedial, medicinal, restorative, salubrious, health-giving, tonic, reparative, corrective, beneficial, good, salutary, recreative.*

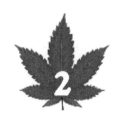

The Endocannabinoid System

Most health-conscience seniors understand the benefit of following a wellness regimen, which includes diet, exercise, and other therapeutic activities. To remain in optimum health, regular visits with a physician coupled with carefully-planned medication regime may also be necessary in order to reduce pain, increase mobility and improve demeanor—among other things. What many seniors are discovering is that cannabis, a once ill-perceived "street drug", may actually be an incredible asset to their over-all health and wellness, as well, especially when used in conjunction with other physician-recommended forms of therapy.

What is Cannabis?

Before delving too deeply into the benefits of cannabis therapeutics, let's look at what cannabis, a.k.a. "marijuana", "weed", "ganja", "bud"—actually is.

While history of cannabis use dates back as far as 440 B.C., the scientific name, *Cannabis Sativa L.*, was first coined in 1753 by botanist Carl Linnaeus. Then, in 1785, a second species of cannabis, *Cannabis Indica,* was introduced by Jean-Baptiste de Lamarck who noted weaker fiber production of the latter but much higher therapeutic value.

Cannabis was widely used to promote physical and spiritual wellness until it became vilified when the newly-established FDA declared drug addiction an epidemic. Cannabis use became a crime with enactment of 1937 Marijuana Tax Act, which was offically repealed by Congress in 1970.

Hemp, which is derived from the same species of *Cannabis Sativa L.*, which is more commonly referred to as "marijuana", differs only in its THC content, which is the main psychoactive component in cannabis and must be less than .03 percent to be considered "hemp". Because of hemp's similarities to the psychoactive cannabis plant, it's cultivation, production and importation was closely regulated until legalization in the Farm Bill of 2018.

Cannabis Therapeutics

Cannabis is much more than a plant. Its chemical composition—and the way those chemicals interact with special receptors throughout the body—suggests that cannabis may be used therapeutically in many beneficial ways. From

Trichromes from the Greek τρίχωμα (trikhō-ma) meaning "hair," are fine outgrowths or appendages on plants, algae, lichens, and certain protists, such as hairs, glandular hairs, scales, and papillae.

pain management to improved demeanor, individual well-being to interpersonal relationships, cannabis's therapeutic value can be a great tool to help seniors achieve balance.

Trichromes

Though the biological composition of hemp and marijuana are similar, it is only female marijuana plants that produce flowers—"buds", and it is the buds alone that contain "trichromes", the sole source of cannabinoids like THC, CBD and others.

High concentration of these crystals is usually a good indication of plant potency and, upon close inspection, can also indicate the maturity of the bud at the time of harvest. For example, buds that are harvested early will have trichromes that are clear and glass-like in appearance.

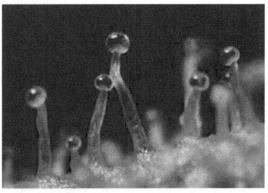

Trichromes are small, mushroom shaped "crystals" that coat the cannabis flower.

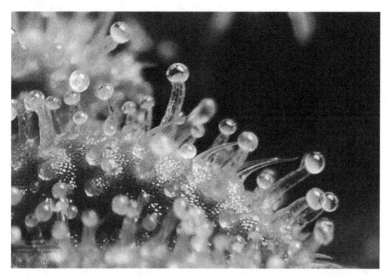

Milky - cloudy trichromes are at their peak cannabinoid production.

Cannabinoids

Cannabis is a complicated plant containing over 400 compounds, of which at least 60 are cannabinoids. They relieve symptoms by attaching to receptors in the brain and in the immune system. Evidence suggests that they

Cannabinoids relieve symptoms by attaching to receptors in the brain and in the immune system.

can improve appetite, reduce muscle pain, quell nasea, reduce inflammation as well as soothe anxiety. However only a few cannabinoids have been identified.

Cannabinoids

THC stands for delta-9-tetrahydrocannibinol and is the cannabinoid that "gets you high." Additonally, it has many medicinal properties: anti-epileptic, anti-inflammatory, anti-depressant, appetite stimulation, and lowering blood pressure.

CBD reduces the psychological effects of the THC in marijuana. CBDs provide more physical body effects such as reducing pain, soothing anxiety, quieting nausa, sedating along with having anti-convulsive, anti-schizophrenic effects.

CBN is similar to THC but with fewer psychological effects. It is produced as THC breaks down within the plant. Higher levels of THC makes CBN effects stronger and is helpful for lowering pressure in the eye (such as with glaucoma), analgesic, anti-seizure.

CBC stands for cannabichromene. Its main job is to enhance the effects of THC, making the strain more potent, with sedative, analgesic and anti-inflammatory effects.

CBG stands for cannabigerol. It has no psychological effects by itself, is thought to be the "parent" to the other cannabinoids and has anti-microbial properties as well as lowering pressure in the eye, and having anti-inflammatory, sedation, and sleep assistance benefits.

The Entourage Effect

The entourage effect is the effect produced from the synergistic interaction of the cannabinoids with other chemicals naturally found in cannabis. Researchers believe that the beneficial effects are greater when cannabis compounds

> *Beneficial effects are greater when cannabis compounds work together.*

work together. Entrouage effect refers to benefits gained from ingesting multiple components of the cannabis plant together instead of ingesting one component at-a-time.

Cannabinoids

	THC	CBD	CBG	CBN	CBC	THCv	CBGA	CGCA	CBCA	THCA
Pain Relief	●	●		●	●		●			
Reduce Seizure		●			●					
Better Sleep				●						
Soothe Anxiety		●								
Low Bld Sugar		●								
Lower Appetite			●							
Kill Bacteria		●	●							
Reduce Nausea	●	●								
Anti-Fugal								●		
Inhibit Tumor		●	●		●					●
Open Artery		●								
Treat Psoriasis		●								
Antipsychotic		●								
Soothe Spasms	●	●						●		●
Up Appetite	●									
Promote Bones		●	●		●	●	●			
Anti-inflamm.		●	●		●		●	●		●

Cannabidiol - CBD

Cannabidiol (CBD) is a non-psychoactive component of cannabis that has a wide range of therapeutic benefits. Preclinical studies suggest that CBD may have therapeutic benefits in the treatment of various conditions, including chronic pain, anxiety, nausea, rheumatoid arthritis, schizophrenia, diabetes, PTSD, alcoholism, strokes and cardiovascular disease, cancer, and other ailments

Dr. Sanjay Gupta, a neurosurgeon, medical professor and Emmy award-winning chief medical correspondent concluded, "The science is there. This isn't anecdotal. We have been terribly and systematically misled for nearly 70 years." Fortunately growing interest in CBD is stimulating needed research.

CBD is available in many different forms. One of them is in a tincture oil. CBD tincture was designed to have the highest CBD absorption rate available. Because tinctures are administered directly under the tongue, the CBD enters the bloodstream much more directly than by any other means so that the action in the body is usually quicker.

CBD holds potential for relieving arthritis pain, which afflicts more than 50 million American. Rheumatoid arthritis is an autoimmune disease in which the immune system attacks the joints, causing inflammation. It most commonly affects the hands and feet and leads to painful, swollen, and stiff joints. Osteoarthritis is a degenerative disease that affects joint cartilage and bones, causing pain and stiffness—most often the hip, knee, and thumb joints.

Researchers believe that CBD brings soothing relief by affecting cannabinoid receptors in the brain and immune system—a view supported by a study with rats that found CBD helped to reduce inflammatory pain by affecting the way that pain receptors respond to stimuli. Another study found that the topical application of CBD relieved inflammation associate with arthritis in rats. However, to date, there is a lack of scientific evidence to prove conclusively that CBD is an effective arthritis treatment for humans. Still it is encouraging

CBD has *low* potential for abuse. It does not contain THC—the chemical that gets marijuana smokers "high" and there are very legitimate medical applications, says Dr. Sanjay Gupta.

Other Cannabinoids

Other common cannabinoids found in the cannabis plant include CBC, which has been shown to reduce pain and inflammation and slow the growth of fungus and bacteria; and CBG, which has been shown to promote bone regeneration and inhibit cancer cell proliferation.

Cannabinoids are an especially important part of the cannabis plant because of the way they interact with our bodies, specifically, their interaction with the endocannabinoid (EC) system. Named after the plant that aided in its discovery, the EC system is composed of a series of receptors located throughout the body. CB1 receptors are located in the brain and spinal cord and affect thought, emotion and memory, while CB2 receptors are found throughout the entire body, including the brain, though to a lesser extent. The density of CB2 receptors in peripheral tissue suggests their activation may have a therapeutic impact on gastrointestinal disorders, autoimmune diseases and chronic or persistent pain.

Though the specific function of the EC system has yet to be determined, research suggests that its purpose is to serve as a mediator between different areas of the body by regulating cellular communication. Cannabinoids may work synergistically to regulate pain, reduce inflammation and decrease stress to speed recovery time.

Researcher Don Wei theorized in the proceedings of the National Academy of Science that cannabis used with friends increases sociability and builds stronger interpersonal connections by causing the brain to release oxytocin, or the "love hormone" upon its consumption.

Indigenous Cannabinoids

Cannabinoids, though first discovered in the cannabis plant, are made in our bodies, as well. Research has revealed that endocannabinoids are created within the body when the need arises and work backwards on presynaptic cells to control the rate at which electrical messages are transmitted throughout the brain and body. Interestingly, though there is a large concentration of CB receptors throughout most of the body, CB receptors seem to be lacking in the part of the brain responsible for heart and lung function, thereby making cannabis-specific overdose unlikely.

Synthetic Cannabinoids

Cannabinoids can also be produced synthetically, though the safety of synthetic cannabinoids is questionable. Acting on the same receptors as other cannabinoids, these "designer drugs" bind completely with CB receptors in the body where they stay attached for a long time—unlike endo- or phytocannabinoids that wear off relatively quickly—and could result in potentially dire consequences like uncontrollable vomiting, seizures and even coma. Unfortunately, because the chemical composition of synthetic cannabinoids is always changing, regulation is extremely difficult. Consumption of synthetic cannabis should always be avoided.

Terpenes

Terpenes are the oils in the trichromes that create flavor and aroma and enhance therapeutic value.

Myrcene:
Therapeutic value: Sedating

Aroma: Earthy, cloves, herbal. Effects: Relaxing. Found in mango, lemongrass, hops & thyme.

Linalool:
Therapeutic value: Anti-anxiety.

Aroma: Floral, citrus, candy. Effects: Sedation, soothes anxiety. Found in lavender.

Limonene:
Therapeutic value: Antiseptic.

Aroma: Citrus. Effects: Stress relief; mood elevation. Found in lemons, oranges, juniper.

Pinene:
Therapeutic value: Anti-inflammatory

Aroma: Pine. Effects: Alertness, increased energy. Found in pine trees, rosemary, sage.

Trans-Caryophyllene:
Therapeutic value: Anti-tumor

Aroma: Pepper, woody, spicy. Effects: Pain relief.

Found in: cotton, black pepper, cloves.

Cannabis Myths

Many are the myths and misconceptions surrounding cannabis and its use. Some conjure cartoonish images of a typical user, such as Cheech and Chong or Willie Nelson. Others maintain that cannabis is a gateway drug to using narcotics like cocaine or heroin. Most of these beliefs are false, born from ignorance or even to intimidate those who are curious about cannabis use and therapeutics.

Myth: Cannabis Is Like Alcohol

That cannabis is like alcohol is often asserted, and makes sense to those who have never actually used cannabis. The truth is that alcohol and cannabis have little in common, with each having unique chemical compositions and very different effects on the human body.

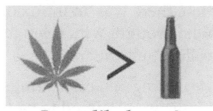

Is pot like booze?

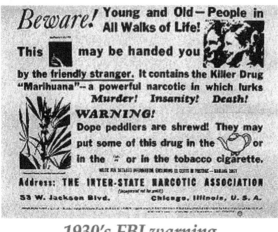

1930's FBI warning.

Most notably, cannabis is a plant and not a "drug", although it is often referred to as such. Alcohol is a drug-like liquid created through fermentation of plants such as wheat, hops, or other grains.

Alcohol travels through the digestive system and is absorbed into the bloodstream through the stomach and the small intestine. It is then metabolized by the liver, which can handle around one ounce of alcohol—about one drink—per hour. When people drink more than their body can metabolize, alcohol builds up in the blood and leads to intoxication.

The myth that the cannabis "high" is similar to alcohol intoxication has its origins during prohibition when drinking alcohol was illegal. At the time there was an influx of Mexican immigration who brought with them a weed they smoked and called "marihuana".

During Senate hearings in the 1930's, marijuana was claimed to cause men—especially

Mexican men—to become aggressive in soliciting sex. The movie *Reefer Madness* portrays this propagandized view. The result was the *Marijuana Tax Act of 1937*, which banned marijuana use and sales. The Act was replaced with the *Controlled Substances Act* in the 1970's, which established "Schedules" for ranking substances according to their dangerousness and potential for addiction. Cannabis was placed in the most restrictive category—Schedule I along with heroin and cocaine.

Alcohol use is associated with many health problems. Drinking too much alcohol—binge drinking—can actually kill the drinker when alcohol builds up in the brain and shuts down heartbeat and respiration. By contrast marijuana can negatively affect the cardiovascular system, increasing heart rate and blood pressure, but people can't fatally overdose on cannabis.

Because seniors often take prescribed medications, drinking alcohol is vastly more dangerous for seniors because alcohol often interacts with other drugs—both illicit and prescription medications—in dangerous

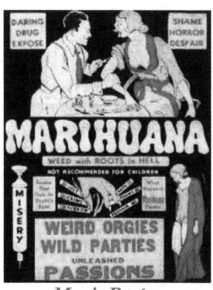

Movie Poster

ways. Using cannabis is much safer for seniors because it doesn't interact with pharmaceuticals.

However, cannabis is still a mood-altering substance and, like alcohol, may lead to impaired judgment or coordination, so it's important to use in a safe and secure environment and abstain from operating a vehicle after use.

Myth: Cannabis Is A Gateway Drug

This myth also took root in the early days of cannabis criminalization. The federal government designated marijuana as a Schedule I substance considered dangerous and addictive, which included drugs like opium and cocaine. The notion was that smoking pot created a kind of appetite for harder drugs.

Most hard drug users began with alcohol and nicotine. Actually most hard drug users began with alcohol and nicotine—often before being of legal age. Marijuana is the first illicit drug most people encounter because it is the most widely used illicit substance. So it is not surprising that most users of "hard" drugs, like heroin, used marijuana first. However, there is no conclusive evidence that the effects of marijuana are causally linked to the subsequent abuse of other illicit drugs.

Research published in *Journal of School Health* concluded that the theory of a gateway drug is not associated with marijuana, and instead points the finger at alcohol that they called the most damaging and socially accepted drug in the world.

"Whether marijuana smokers go on to use other illicit drugs depends more on social factors like being exposed to stress and being unemployed, not so much whether they smoked a joint in the eighth grade," explained Dr. Karen Van Gundy, associate professor of psychology at the University of New Hampshire. "Because underage smoking and alcohol use typically precede marijuana use, marijuana is not the most common, and is rarely the first illicit drug used."

Myth: Cannabis Causes Cognitive Decline

The stereotype of the "forgetful stoner" is often seen on TV and in movies, and there is some truth in the connection between cannabis use and memory loss. However, there is further evidence that shows cannabis therapeutics promotes cognitive function. Research by Jiang, et.al., published in the *Journal of Clinical Investigation* found that the active ingredients in cannabis promotes cell growth in the brain, also called "neurogenesis". Furthermore, those new brain cells may link to a reduction in anxiety and depression.

Cannabis therapeutics shows promise in the treatment of Alzheimer's disease. Researchers

Currasi, et.al., reported in *Aging and Mechanisms of Disease* that the cannabinoid, THC, promotes the removal of plaque in the brain, a common feature of Alzheimer's. Additionally, they found that cannabis has anti-inflammatory properties and helps protect neurons in the brain.

"It is reasonable to conclude that there is a therapeutic potential of cannabinoids for the treatment of Alzheimer's disease," wrote David Schubert, senior researcher and a professor at Salk Institute for Biological Studies.

Cannabis may also be helpful in boosting creativity. According to research conducted at University of California at Berkeley Medical School, the active ingredients in the plant stimulate the frontal lobe of the brain, which is responsible for innovation and divergent thinking. This can promote a better quality of life and assist people in engaging in new activities.

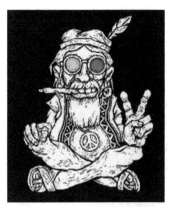

Stoner stereotype.

Myth: Cannabis Is Only For "Stoners"

It's not just college kids and hip 20-somethings that engage in cannabis use. While the media may portray the typical marijuana user as young and silly, the truth is that there really is no "typical" user. People of all

ages—from children to senior citizens—use cannabis for a variety of reasons. This may include both
medical and recreational use; a senior may smoke
marijuana to relax or to soothe pain. As research
into the benefits of cannabis continue, more treatments for a variety of ailments are expected in the
coming years.

The number of seniors trying cannabis is increasing rapidly. Many seniors had experience with
cannabis in their younger days, while other seniors
are trying it for the first
time. In fact, people ages 55
and older is now the fast-
est-growing demographic
of pot users in the country,
with marijuana use up 53
percent. From 2013 to 2014,
the number of seniors using
pot increased from 2.8 million to 4.3 million, according
to a report released by CBS
News. Pot is rapidly becom-
ing the pill alternative as seniors look for an alternative to pharmaceutical medications, especially powerful opioid painkillers and sleep aides.

© Ljupeo Smokovski

*Pot is becoming the
"pill alternative".*

Get the Facts

Discuss cannabis with family, friends, and quali-
fied professionals to get information to decide if
using cannabis may be beneficial for you.

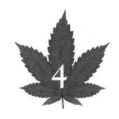

Routes into the Bloodstream

Medicines work in a variety of ways depending on the purpose for which they are taken. We may take medicine to relieve pain, to fight disease, or to supplement a deficiency as examples.

In addition to deciding what medicine to take, there is the form by which a medication is taken. Medicines can enter the body in many different ways, including through an inhaler, a skin patch, a pill, a hypodermic needle, and even through the rectum. Once the medicines are inside your body they move into the blood stream, then into organs and tissues to produce or induce effects.

Understanding how medicines work in your body can help you learn how to best use cannabis therapeutics to address your specific concerns.

Seniors wanting to use cannabis to uplift mood, reduce pain, or for other reasons need to weight the pros and cons of using cannabis as well as considering which method of use is best for them. As an unique being, "you" are central to these decisions. Cannabis therapeutics is not simply "popping a pill," because the plant's cannabinoids interact with your unique psychology and bodily chemistry as the compounds get into the blood to manifest the beneficial effects.

Injection

Injection is the fastest route into the bloodstream, because a syringe or needle puts the substance directly into the blood. Because cannabis is not water-soluble, the injection route is not available for cannabis. Morphine and similar narcotics are water-soluble and can be injected, which lead them to supplant cannabis as a medicine early in the 20th century because the dangers of opiates were not fully revealed until decades later.

Inhalation

Inhaling cannabis smoke from a marijuana cigarette or "joint," a pipe, or water pipe or "bong" is the traditional method for using it. Those enjoying recreational cannabis tend to favor inhalation because it is fast in producing cannabis effects. When inhaled, the smoke is drawn into the lungs, which enables the active components to quickly enter the bloodstream so they can be carried to the brain. In the brain there are endogenous cannabinoid receptors that accept the active components of cannabis to enable them to do their magic.

Consider what happens when smoking tobacco cigarettes. Nicotine—the addictive drug in tobacco smoke—has a rapid effect on the smoker. In the same way, active chemicals in cannabis, like THCs, CBCs and CBDs, which are not considered addictive, travel into the bloodstream to effect their therapeutic benefits.

Joint

A plus of inhalation is that the active chemicals in the cannabis smoke travel quickly through the lungs into the blood. Many report that they experience nearly instant effects when inhaling cannabis. Such speed is especially important when seeking to soothe pain, for example.

Ease of titration is a less-recognized but an equally important benefit of inhalation. Titration is a process of inhaling small amounts until you have had enough cannabis. Then you stop smoking for a while. When smoking cannabis for pain, for example, you may sense an easing of the pain and

A benefit of inhalation is the ease of titration—of deciding when you have inhaled enough cannabis to stop smoking for the time being.

then can "pass the dubbie"—after a while,
you may smoke a little more to maintain the pain relief—while relaxing with friends in the evening.

The above   example
illustrates another   benefit of
inhaling canna-   bis. Chemicals in
cannabis encour-   age conviviality and
relaxation, which is   additionally encouraged
when "passing a pipe" then taking "a hit" when
it circles around to you. Social interaction is encouraged by such cannabis "rituals"— as socializing is itself healing. Cannabis is a "mind/body"
therapeutic that can help reduce the social isolation and loneliness many seniors experience

Eating

"Edibles" are foods containing cannabinoids.
Eating is a popular method for getting the soothing chemicals in cannabis into the bloodstream.
When eaten, the cannabinoids are absorbed
through the stomach, which is a different route
from the one taken when cannabinoids are inhaled into the lungs. Like all foods, edibles containing cannabinoids go to the stomach where the
cannabis-laced food is digested and moved into
the intestines where cannabinoids are absorbed
into the bloodstream, then travel to the liver for
processing, and is then moved by the blood to
cannabinoid receptors.

Even though we use the digestive process every day, most of us don't think about digestion. With cannabis therapeutics it is important to understand how cannabinoids work when digested. Digestion is a slow process. Eating cannabis edibles can take two hours or even longer to have a perceivable effect.

When learning to use cannabis edibles, the risk for seniors is that it is easy to eat too much. The mistake is not solely a matter of misjudging the strength of the cannabinoids in the food, but being impatient due to not understanding the process. People who are naive about edibles often expect to experience an effect quickly—like in 15 minutes, which is rarely long enough. When inexperienced seniors make this mistake they may eat a second or even third serving of the cannabis-laced food before their body has digested the first serving so that they eat too much.

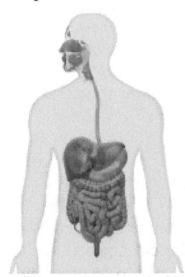

In eating, when the cannabis effects finally "come on", they cannot be easily stopped. So the effects become stronger and stronger for hours, resulting to unpleasant experiences such as

Edibles enter through the stomach.

spasms and other gastrointestinal distress, confusion
and anxiety—even panic.
The effects can be so distressing that people worry
that they are dying and are

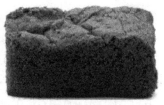

Brownie

taken to the emergency room in an ambulance—
where little can be done, except to comfort the person until the effects of the cannabinoids wear off.

However, a major benefit of eating rather than
inhaling cannabis is that the effects, while taking
a long time to "come on", they also continue for
a long time. Many seniors find this benefit especially helpful in managing pain and stress. A
side beneficial effect is slowing down, which can
reduce anxiety. It is from this effect that so-called
"pot heads" are considered "mellow". "Hey, mellow out, Man. Stop and smell the flowers!" Developing patience is a benefit for seniors who use
edibles as a mind/body therapeutic.

Absorption Through Skin

Most people think the lungs are the body's largest
organ when the largest organ is the skin—while
the lungs are the largest internal organ in the body.
The skin provides a non-invasive route for absorption of cannabinoids into the bloodstream because
it does not go through the digestion system.

Like other substances administered transdermally, cannabinoids pass through seven cell layers of the epidermis into the lower skin layer, the dermis—where they enter the bloodstream. Then the cannabinoids are carried in the blood to the endogenous cannabinoid receptors in the brain through which they have their effects.

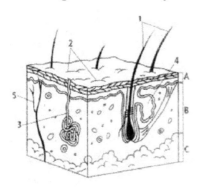

Layers of epidermis.

There's increasing interest in use of skin as a route for absorption of cannabis and other therapeutics. For example, pain patches are already used by seniors. Medicinal patches are small adhesive-backed pads saturated with medicine in the middle. Cannabinoid therapeutics use the same route as that taken pharmaceutical narcotic patches—through the epidermis, the outer skin layers, to the dermis, the inner part of the skin into the bloodstream.

Sublingual Absorption

Another fast route for cannabinoids to get into the bloodstream, without inhaling is sublingual cannabis therapeutics. This involves placing a cannabinoid-containing preparation—a tincture—under the tongue for sublingual administration. There are many tiny blood vessels in the area under the tongue called capillaries. Through capillaries the cannabinoids can directly enter into the bloodstream. However, caution is needed to not swallow the tincture, which will take the cannabinoids into the digestion system, which is much slower.

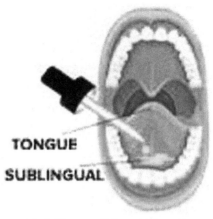

TONGUE

SUBLINGUAL

Sublingual is under the tongue

Seniors who seek to get effects quickly because of an acute attack of arthritic pain, for example, find sublingual cannabis especially useful because of the speed of getting relief. Because the cannabinoids do not go through the digestive system, they are not metabolized by the liver, so that a lower dose may be effective, than when using edibles. Because the cannabinoids enter the blood directly through the capillaries, sublingual administration is especially useful for seniors experiencing difficulty in swallowing.

Suppositories

A little known method of application, but one with a number of benefits, is the suppository. As discussed earlier, cannabis edibles can take as long as two hours for the medicinal effects to be noticed. And there is potential that the previous

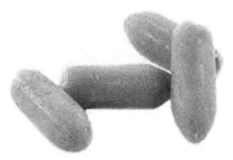

Interest in cannabis suppositories is increasing.

meal may effect the rate at which the medicine takes effect. By contrast most people begin to notice effects of a cannabis suppository in ten to fifteen minutes after insertion. This is because suppositories and enemas inserted into the bowel through the anal opening is usually swift acting due to the large surface area of the bowel that is packed with blood vessels, so absorbing the cannabinoids can be very quickly.

While there is limited research, interest in cannabis suppositories is increasing. Numerous anecdotal accounts suggest that rectal administration of suppositories may provide the most effective way for some to take in the cannabis therapeutics. Due to the large surface area available for absorption and the speed in which the cannabinoids are absorbed, using suppositories may be a suitable route when there are restrictions on oral ingestion such as before and after surgery. Other cases where suppositories may be helpful includes people with gastrointestinal difficulties, an impaired jaw or throat or whose nausea and vomiting prevent effective oral application.

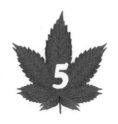

How to Use Cannabis

Many who enjoy cannabis have transitioned beyond the traditional joint to other methods of ingestion. Alternative options for ingestion are often favored because they tend to be slightly healthier, somewhat easier to prepare than joints, pipes and other conventional smoking methods and more discrete.

Decarbing Cannabis

Decarboxylation is a process of preparing the cannabis to be most available for use. To release the cannabis's psychoactive effects, it must be dried, aged—and "decarboxylated" or heated. Applying heat to dried bud triggers fascinating chemical reactions in the plant where the plant compounds are transformed into cannabinoid acids into a form usable by the body with heat. It is important to go low and slow in temperature with heat at about 212 degrees for 100 minutes.

Cannabinoids are chemicals found in the cannabis plant that bind to receptors in the body to produce therapeutic effects. Sometimes decarboxylation is called "activating" or "decarbing".

The primary psychoactive compound in cannabis is delta9-tetrahydrocannabinol (THC). THC is what causes the "high". But, not much THC is found on a live, growing marijuana plant, if any at all. What is found instead is another compound called THCA, which is short for tetrahydrocannabinolic acid. THCA is *not* psychoactive and will not get the user high. In order to feel the mind-altering effects of cannabis, THCA must be transformed into psychoactive THC, which is done by appling a little heat.

Putting a lighter to a joint or placing cannabis in the oven causes a bit of chemistry as one compound is converted into another—turning an otherwise non-psychoactive plant into a psychoactive one. Specifically, a "carboxyl group" is removed from the acid form of THC. Hence the term *"De-carboxylation"*. Without that carboxyl group, THC is then able to freely bind to cell receptors in the brain and body.

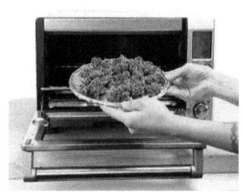

***Decarbing activates
cannabinoids***

Inhale Cannabis

Cannabis can be burned or baked and then consumed by smoking or inhaling vapor. Some
prefer vaping pens while others are
partial to joints made with
rolling paper, pipes and bongs
for inhalation.

When smoking cannabis in a pipe or joint, the
plant material is burned, which yields smoke to
be inhaled. Alternatively, when using a vaporizer, the cannabis is *baked* in a miniature oven-like
compartment in the device. Cannabis will not
burn unless it is dried and aged. When moisture
is removed from cannabis it is ready to smoke.
Heated cannabis creates pain-relieving compounds during the decarboxylation process in
which cannabinoid acids are transformed to a
form the body can use for pain relief.

Without the initial decarbing, the user will
receive little to no therapeutic benefit from the
plant. The application of heat turns tetrahydrocannabinolic acid into delta9-tetrahydrocannab-
inol (THC) to produce pain-relieving effects.
As smokers light and puff on the cannabis they
are acting like a kind of chemist transforming a
compound into an enhanced version to produce
amazing physical and mental benefits.

Proper Dosing

To use cannabis therapeutics effectively the smoker must use the proper dosage to reap the positive effects from the compounds in the plant. A small dose will not make much of an impact on pain or mental state. An overly large dose has the potential to trigger uber-euphoric feelings and disorientation.

It can take upwards of 10 minutes for smoked cannabis to produce perceived effects because it takes an amount of time for the compounds to reach the blood stream and produce the intended effects. A couple of factors come into play when determining how quickly cannabis effects impact the body. Different cannabis strains produce varied results, with many strains requiring mere minutes to produce the intended effects while others can take 10 minutes or longer. How the strain is cured, harvested, and stored makes a difference because THC can degrade into THCv, for example. THCv boosts energy and suppresses appetite, but doesn't produce the high characteristic of THC.

Smoking Pros and Cons

The benefits of smoking are many.   Pain-relieving benefits come on quickly when smoking as compared to eating cannabis—edibles. Pipes and rolling papers are cheap. Add in the fact that smoking is an enjoyable, and somewhat nostalgic process, and it is easy to see why so many people prefer to smoke their cannabis.

There are a few drawbacks to smoking cannabis. Smoking produces a strong odor that can seep to nearby rooms. If the smoke is not passed through a water pipe, the patient will be subjected to excessive carcinogenic properties. Also, preparing the smoking device takes more time than the comparably simple ingestion of a pre-made edible, like a cookie or brownie.

Vaporizing Cannabis

Inhaling vaporized cannabis yields more powerful effects. Vaping tends to boost the potency of cannabis, generating a purer flavor with minimal to no odor. Vaporizers bake cannabis in a miniature oven-like compartment in the device rather than burn it. The baking process combined with the absence of rolling papers means that the user is not inhaling carcinogens. Compared to having to roll a joint, which takes some skill, many

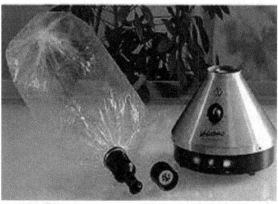

Valcano vaporizer—vapor is captured in the plastic bag.

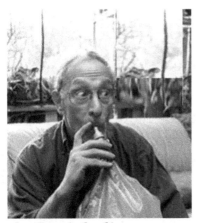

Senior inhaling vapor.

prefer vaping, which is easier—and probably more healthy, too.

Cannabis smoking can create respiratory problems. Cannabis vaporization is a technique aimed at suppressing irritating respiratory toxins by heating cannabis to a temperature where active cannabinoid vapors form, but below the point of combustion where smoke and associated toxins are produced. Vaporizers heat cannabis to release active cannabinoids, but remain cool enough to avoid the smoke and toxins associated with combustion. Vaporized cannabis should create fewer respiratory symptoms than smoked cannabis.

Vaping does have a few negatives. Vaporizing equipment is more expensive than smoking equipment. Cannabis concentrates used in a vape tend to be more difficult to acquire than the plant material. Because vaping pens and vaporizers must be recharged, the device may not be ready to use when wanted.

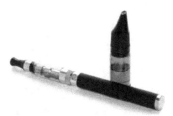

Cannabis oil vaporizor.

Duration of the "High"

Inhaled cannabis has the potential to disorient peoples who consume a large dosage. This can be avoided by starting off with a single hit, then relaxing for about 10 minutes before taking another puff. You will likely feel a little euphoria—feel good—and pain relief. This "high" has the potential to last an hour to upwards of six hours. The length of the high hinges on an array of factors such as the smoker's metabolic rate, the type of strain consumed, the potency of the strain and the frequency of consumption.

Eating Cannabis

As with smoking, cannabis should be decarboxilated before consumption. This "toasting" of cannabis allows the plant's psychoactive properties to manifest for pain relief and feelings of euphoria. Always decarb the dried cannabis before ingesting it by lightly toasting for 10-20 minutes in an oven below 300 degrees Fahrenheit. Keeping the oven 300 degrees ensures that the cannabinoids do not burn.

Larger buds should be broken up to facilitate decarbing. The length of time required for decarbing hinges on the freshness of the cannabis as well as the amount. Fresh cannabis requires a longer decarbing time.

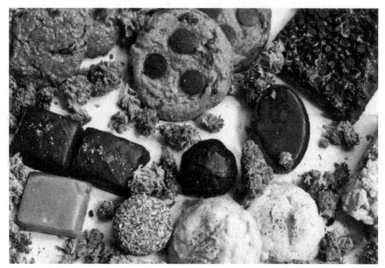

Edibles come in dozens of delicious varieties.
Always start with a small piece.

Proper Dosing

When first experimenting with an edible, start out
with a very low dose. If you buy a cookie at a dispensary, it is a good idea to start of with half of it.
Notice how you are effected. Be patient. Look for
subtle effects. Use your self-observation to make a
small adjustment in the amount you eat [more or
less] next time.

When eaten, cannabis has the potential to trigger ecstatic feeling and to lessen physical pain and
mental distress. But eating needs to be approached
slowly with a small dose in the first several uses.
Set aside a few hours for the first experience—perhaps a whole day in some cases—to arrange for
responsibilities such as driving and child care.

Skin Absorption

Topical cannabis products are applied directly to the skin and used to reduce local pain and skin irritations, but don't produce euphoric highs. Cannabinoids must have the assistance of "carrier agents", such as oleic acid and dimethyl sulfoxide, to be effective. If a carrier agent is not present, the topical agent won't pass through the blood brain barrier. Check the label of topical cannabis creams, gels and patches to ensure they feature a carrier agent and have been decarbed before processing lest the desired therapeutic effects not be achieved.

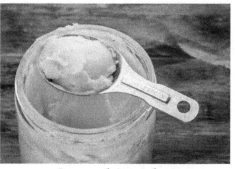

Cannabis salve.

Cannabinoids applied topically interact with the skin and nerves locally to reduce pain and inflammation. Topical cannabis products can mitigate skin disorders. Give the topical ointment at least 20 minutes to work its magic. Conversely, transdermal cannabis products penetrate deeply to provide full-body pain relief with the gradual release of cannabinoids into the bloodstream across eight to 12 hours.

Always follow the recommended dosage with topical ointments as with other ingestion methods. For local relief, apply the ointment to the area two or three times per day. For full-body relief, use a transdermal dose at 2 mg. Note: a 10 mg transdermal dose is about 80 mg. of edibles.

Sublingual Absorption

Sublingual absorption is a highly effective method of consuming cannabis that requires minimal preparation and equipment. Sublingual use of cannabis is easy. A tincture dose is applied with a dropper under the tongue. Cannabis used to make tinctures as well as other edible cannabis products requires decarboxylation as described earlier.

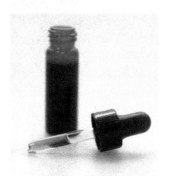

A drop of cannabis tinture is placed under tongue.

Some "edibles" are coated in tincture and work well when administered under the tongue or between the gums and cheek. The dose for first-time sublingual cannabis use is 10 mg, which can be increased as you becomes accustomed to the tincture's effects

Experiment

Because each method varies so much in terms of potency, speed of onset, duration and effects on the body, some methods may be better—or worse—than others for you depending on your desired effects and outcome.

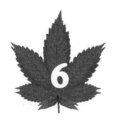

Therapeutic Strains

Cannabis Sativa L. consists of three species: indica, sativa and ruderalis. The cannabinoid profile of each species differs, which alters their therapeutic qualities. Years of careful breeding of these species has resulted in countless strains with unique cannabinoid profiles and other defining characteristics. These varying types offer different effects, so it is important for seniors to research and personally test strains for individual therapeutic use.

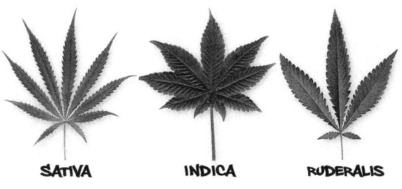

SATIVA   INDICA   RUDERALIS

Leaves of three strains of Cannabis Sativa L.

Cannabis Indica

Indica may be the most prolific strain, due its dominance in several types of cannabis plants. Known

Indica is the most prolific strain and is used for pain relief, anxiety, and good sleep.

to provide more of a "body buzz", this strain is optimal for relaxation and sedation. It is often used for pain relief, anxiety and promoting sleep. Indica is sometimes referred to as "in-da-couch" due to its mellowing effects. Many people prefer to use indica strains at night in order to wind down for sleeping.

Cannabis strains with indica dominance typically have buds larger and more compact with less "ornamental pigment" characteristic of their origin in the Hindu Kush Mountain Range and how many indica strains have been named Kush. The original classification of Cannabis indica was made by French biologist Jean-Baptiste Lamarck in 1785. Lamarck observed that certain marijuana plants from India were intoxicating and could be made into hashish. But traditional hemp crops, which were more common in Europe, had no mind-altering effect.

Indica strains are a common choice for indoor growing because they grow smaller and mature more quickly than other types. Pure indica strains usually finish around 8 weeks of flowering, while pure sativa strains usually finish around 12-14 weeks. People who are growing a few plants for personal consumption find indicas easy to manage, even without professional cannabis grow knowledge.

Cannabis Sativa

Sativa strains tend to cause a more profound cerebral experience, helping to increase energy, alertness, creativity and sociability. Often called "Haze", sativa tends to be used during the day to promote motivation and clarity. Fans of sativas enjoy being able to remain vigorous yet relaxed at the same time. While sativas are a popular choice, finding strains that are 100% sativa-dominant may be difficult due to the development of cross-breeding.

Sativa flowers are smaller "popcorn" shaped buds with more adverse coloration. Ornamental colors like purple, red and dark green help protect the buds from strong UV rays, the evolutionary result of its origins near the equator. Sativas are often reserved for outdoor gardens because of their large size and later maturi-

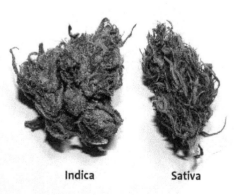

Indica   Sativa

Indica and sativa buds.

ty rate. Some sativa strains yield plants that grow up to 25 feet tall. This may mean a bigger yield but the maintenance definitely requires more work.

Strains that are sativa-dominant may contain high levels of THC that can cause paranoia in some people. These effects can be mediated with cannabidiol (CBD), a non-psychoactive cannabinoid found in cannabis. CBD is mostly derived from hemp and has shown efficacy in alleviating anxiety. It has been touted as a potential therapy for epilepsy and other seizure disorders. CBD products such as oils, tinctures, and edibles are good to have on hand just in case the THC causes discomfort.

Sativa v Indica

Energy	Couch-Potato
Stimulating	Chilling
Head High	Body
Cerebral	Appetite
Uplifting	Relaxing
Creativity	Sleep Aid
Focus	Soothes Pain
Anti-Depression	Anti-Anxiety

Cannabis Ruderalis

Often considered the forgotten cannabis strain, ruderalis is rarely commercially produced because of its low yield and low THC content. However, it has significantly higher amounts of CBD, which makes it the preferred strain for certain therapies. Producers of CBD-infused products often use ruderalis in breeding for a more efficient source of the cannabinoid. The plant is easy to grow and is a great choice for beginners.

Cannabis ruderalis has adapted to extreme climates such as Northern Europe, Northern Russia and Canada. These regions have short growing seasons, typically around three months. Normal cannabis indica/sativa simply can't grow properly in cold climates with short summers. Cannabis ruderalis can grow in extremely short

Ruderalis strains, while lesser known, have high levels of CBD and are becoming more prevalent as a therapy option due its efficacy in quelling seizures and arthritis.

growing seasons because the plant automatically flowers upon maturation. In contrast, indicas and sativas are autotrophic plants and require a careful light schedule to flower. Breeders may crossbreed with ruderalis strains and sell the resulting "autoflowering" seeds at an often increased price.

Hybrid Strains

The majority of commercially available strains on the market today are some sort of indica/sativa hybrid. Breeders have meticulously crossbred different strains over many generations to develop high-quality cannabis strains of varying cannabinoid levels, flavor profiles, physical characteristics and psychological effects. For example, a hybrid may be created that has the cerebral effects of a sativa while also offering the relaxation that indica tends to induce.

Many custom hybrid strains have been developed to achieve certain goals. For example, a CBD-heavy strain called Charlotte's Web was specially created for a young girl—Charlotte—who was afflicted with an extreme form of epilepsy. After Charlotte responded well, use of CBD for seizure disorders has grown with considerable success. Other custom hybrid creations meant to aid a variety of ailments in order to offer the most efficient cannabis therapy possible.

Thanks to centuries of custom cannabis breeding, there are thousands of cannabis strains available, allowing consumers to "shop around" for the perfect strain for their needs and desired experience. Discussing the potential effects of various strains with a professional at a medical marijuana dispensaries will help to determine which strains with which to experiment. Hybrids are an opportunity to explore what multiple strains may do, both physically and psychologically.

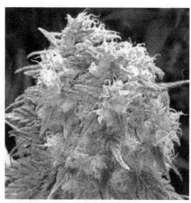

Breeders are creating amazing hybrids.

The three main strain types of cannabis—sativa, indica, and ruderalis—affect the body in varying ways. Indicas are great for relaxation, pain relief, and insomnia while sativas tend to increase energy. Ruderalis strains, while lesser known, have high levels of CBD and are becoming more prevalent as a therapy option due its efficacy in aiding certain ailments such as seizure disorders and arthritis. There are many hybrids that contain multiple types of strains, so it is important to get as much information as possible before moving forward. Experiment with different strains to determine which works best for you.

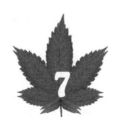

7

Tailor Your Therapeutics

Each of us is different, with unique bodies, minds, and experiences. Anti-depressants, sleeping pills, and other "heavy" pharmaceuticals tend to be crude treatments applied to everyone across the board. Pop a pill and the distress soon goes away without any further efforts by the person in distress or the physician.

The pharmaceutical does not "cure" the distress, but rather masks it—blots it out for a short time. Then the distress returns. Pop another pill to turn it off again. Soon it takes more pills to get the same relief. The risk of dependency is virtually 100%. And the treat-

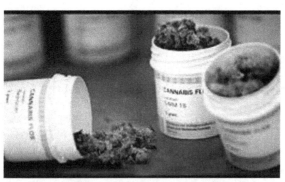

Cannabis therapeutics works differently from pharmaceuticals.

ment, wherein we passively pop powerful "blot out" pills, tends to exacerbate feelings of being a helpless victim of the distressing condition from which we're suffering.

Using cannabis as a therapeutic to help relieve the distress of depression, anxiety, pain, and other conditions works differently. The cannabinoids interact with our unique bodily system in different ways and to different degrees. The effects of using cannabis are subtle, it soothes and relieves the distress. Cannabis does not turn distress off—click, like a light switch. For that you need a narcotic, with which comes all kinds of negative side trips. Because cannabis effects are subtle, they can be missed—especially at first for the new user. Using cannabis therapeutically takes learning how.

Self-Awareness

An important aspect of using cannabis therapeutics is self-awareness—noticing and studying how and where you experience the distress. Then, using a small amount of cannabis, generally by smoking or eating, and then again noticing and studying how you are effected.

With any change program, first changes are small and easy to dismiss. But in dismissing, the change program is stifled. Noticing early small progress is important for motivation to continue

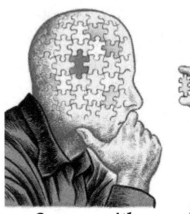

Success with cannabis therapeutics begins with self-awarenss.

with the therapeutic program. But when pain, or anxiety, or depression is so strong, even overpowering, it is difficult to discern a small change for the positive.

So an important component of cannabis therapeutics is detecting and focusing upon improvement. The old glass is half full rather than half empty approach.

You've got to see the positive to focus on it. Here's how. In order to detect change, whether small or large, you must have something to compare it to—a baseline. If you go out and say, "Hey, it is a warm day", you are making a relative statement: today is warmer than most days. "Most days" is the basis of comparison. The comparison tool is called a "baseline".

Establish a Baseline

The first step in using cannabis as a therapeutic is to establish a baseline for your distress level. Let's say you are suffering from high anxiety and feeling nervous and stressed much of the time. That is too vague to be useful. You need to quantify your level of anxiety to establish a baseline. Imagine a scale from 1 to 9, with 9 being extremely anxious and 1 being not anxious.

Do this now. Stop what you are doing and focus your attention on your anxiety—or depression or pain level. Notice the anxiety. Don't judge it or try to change it. Just notice the anxious feelings—the sensations. Where do you feel the anxiety? How does the anxiety feel?

Now using the scale from 1 to 9, rate your level of anxiety. It is a good idea to write down in a small notebook or journal the date and time with your rating and what you were doing right before stopping to rate your anxiety. Repeat this process a couple of times a day for a couple of days and always write down your ratings and a note as to what you were doing right *before* rating yourself.

Study your "data". What are your ratings? Are they wide ranging—different ratings each time, or do they tend to be at the same level. If the ratings ranged widely, look at what you were doing right *before* the rating. For

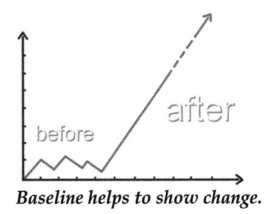

Baseline helps to show change.

example, you may have been cleaning house, or haggling with your daughter, or talking on the phone to a friend, as examples. Is there any relationship between those activities and the level of the anxiety ratings? If you do find a relationship, this is valuable information, pointing to potential anxiety triggers and ways you might be able to use cannabis therapeutics to handle them. Suppose, for example, you see that when you speak to your daughter on the phone you have high anxiety ratings. In this case, you may inhale a small "hit" of cannabis before calling your daughter as an anxiety intervention.

Assessing Change

After you've established your baseline through such self-study over a few days, the next step is to assess effects of the cannabis intervention. Following the example with inhaling a little cannabis before making the call to your daughter, during the call—after you "medicated"—you would focus in on yourself and your anxiety level a couple of times during and then after the call to rate your anxiety level. Write the rating down in your journal, along with notes about the conversation with your daughter.

Using cannabis takes learning, unlike when using pharmaceuticals. The effects are subtle. It is less that the anxiety or pain or depression "goes away", but a process of your mind drifting away from the distress, of your mind letting it go. You are still aware that there is a sense of pain, but it is no longer "painful". This is quite different from what happens with taking narcotic drugs, which tend to blot out your awareness and anesthetize you sometimes to the point of unconsciousness.

There is a famous video from the 1970's played to most psychology students of the time wherein a man named Jack Schwartz was being interviewed and filmed as he takes a sharpened knitting needle and, while describing his experience, proceeds to push the needle into and through the muscle of his upper arm. Viewers can see the indent in the skin as the needle goes in and on the other side as the needle comes out with a drop of blood. While doing this Schwartz tells the interviewer that he is over in the corner, watching himself push the needle into "an arm"—not his arm. He shows no pain in the process.

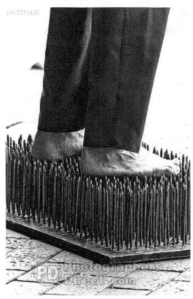

Man stands on nails without pain.

This is a kind of mental gymnastics beyond most of us. This same process is in operation with yogis laying on a bed of nails. The nails are digging into their skin, but they show no sign of pain. And curiously when getting up, they have few marks on their backs. With Schwartz, after he pulls the needles out—with the skin sticking to it and pulling like a small tent, there is at most one to two drops of blood and the wound closes up and disappears. The Schwartz video is available on YouTube and worth watching.

What Schwartz demonstrates with the needle is that much of pain—depression, anxiety—is controlled by the mind and by attention to it. Pain gets more intense when focused upon. When we can "get our mind off of it" for a few minutes we experience

> *Much of pain—depression, anxiety—is controlled by the mind and by your attention to it.*

a bit of relief. The cannabis high is similar to this process. It is not so much as being "high"—as it is of the mind drifting off of worries and hassles and off of aches and pains, to another place and in the process we experience relief. Cannabis helps us in the mind-drifting process. But it also requires learning, which is accelerated by seeing and feeling the effects—by getting feedback.

Acknowledge Progress

By rating the degree of distress before and after using cannabis therapeutics you create a way of seeing a change—even when *very* small. It is important to refine your self-sensing to notice—feel—*small improvements*, which otherwise you may miss. If you don't see your progress, you will likely get discouraged and give up learning to use cannabis therapeutics. For example, when your self-rating after inhaling cannabis shows a *small* movement in the desired direction—i.e., a small soothing of anxiety—as com-

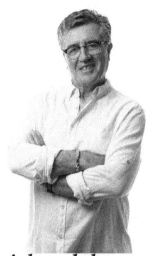

Kues1

Acknowledge your progress especially in the beginning.

pared to your baseline—how you felt *before* using the cannabis, then you are likely to be encouraged—motivated—by your progress. Pat yourself on the back for *small improvements*.

It is important to focus on the positive change, not the negative, and to *actively tell yourself* that your efforts are working and you are making progress in getting control of your anxiety (pain, depression, etc.).

Feelings of pride in beginning to control runaway anxiety, as in this example, without the use of heavy pharmaceuticals is empowering and accelerates the learning process—learning how to use cannabis therapeutics.

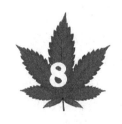

Senior Opioid Epidemic

An emerging threat to the health and longevity of senior citizens has been identified. It lurks in the medicine cabinets of millions of seniors: opioid medicines. Opioids include opiates, like morphine, as well as powerful but very commonly prescribed synthetic drugs like hydrocodone, oxycodone and fentanyl. While drug dependency and abuse have long been shortening the lives of the nation's youth and younger adults, prescription opioid abuse has now become a silent scourge of seniors across the country. But perhaps there's a novel way to solve this problem in society's more accepting attitude toward cannabis. Could cannabis hold the key to solving the senior opioid epidemic?

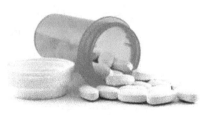

Seniors are at risk.

According to a 2015 study by the Substance Abuse and Mental Health Services Administration (SAMHSA) and U.S.

Department of Health and Human Services (HHS), a third of chronic prescription drug users are over

For senior citizens, opioid abuse usually starts with a legitimate prescription for chronic pain.

65, while being just 13 percent of the population. Research out of Towson University found a 78 percent jump from 2006 to 2012 in ER visits for misuse or overdose of prescription or illegal drugs. Half of these visits were made by individuals age 75 and older. A startling 11 percent of those cases involved opioids.

In 2009, the American Geriatrics Society reversed years of policy in updating their pharmacological guidelines to no longer recommend over-the-counter pain meds (such as NSAIDs or COX-2 inhibitors) before prescribing opioids for chronic pain to older patients—which hastened the rise in opioid use.

Meanwhile, the Agency for Healthcare Research and Quality shows rates of adults between the age of 45 and 85 being hospitalized for opioid use to have risen by 500 percent since 1993. The numbers are stark, and show a nation in the throes of an epidemic. In response the Centers for Disease Control and Prevention issued an array of recommended guidelines for the prescription of opioids. This is a response to the fact that opioid prescriptions have gone up fourfold since 1999. It is quite troubling that 40 people die each day as a result of opioid overdoses.

Younger people have traditionally found their way to opiate addiction through recreational use, leading them to seek out prescriptions when supply becomes an issue. For senior citizens, opioid abuse usually starts from a legitimate prescription for chronic pain. Within just five days some users can become dependent. This leads to seniors, who tend to have better health insurance, to frequently seek out more than one doctor, stacking prescriptions for different pains, causing their tolerance to rapidly increase.

As tolerance to the opioids grows, higher doses and new prescriptions are required, all the while the pain relievers are not actually treating the underlying pain, merely masking it. This is an underlying cause of opioid addiction, and before long, it is unclear to the user whether they need the opioid more for the pain of their injury, or for their addiction to avoid withdrawal pain.

> *The pain relieving opiods are not actually treating the underlying pain, but merely masking it.*

Soon functioning begins to visibly decline, but often with seniors the symptoms of this decline are assumed to be fatigue, dementia, "senior moments," or just the regular signs of aging. Accidental overdosing can often exacerbate this, as it may be difficult to keep complicated dosing schedules in order across several different prescriptions.

Seniors Becoming Addicted

The unfortunate truth is that a growing number of seniors are becoming addicted to opioids, some to the point of life threatening overdoses. Seniors are particularly vulnerable to opioid side effects and subsequent falls and missteps due to their increasingly fragile bodies. According to the health education informational network Family Doctor, senior citizens in the United States consume about 33 percent of the nation's prescription drugs. This is a shocking statistic considering the fact that senior citizens represent merely 13 percent of the total population. Though many seniors truly need opioids to manage pain, it is clear that doctors give prescriptions too freely to

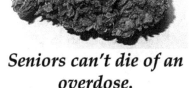

Seniors can't die of an overdose.

seniors and a growing number have developed unhealthy dependency.

Upwards of 15 percent of seniors who seek medical assistance are abusing prescription drugs. According to Johns Hopkins Medical School, there will be 2.7 million Americans over the age of 50 abusing prescription drugs by 2020. This represents a 190 percent increase from the 910,000 of the same age cohorts who abused prescription drugs in 2001. Part of the cause of seniors' dependency on opioids is that seniors can access drugs with ease. Many seniors have more than one doctor who prescribes them medication. In some instances, seniors intentionally visit with numerous doctors and use different pharmacies to procure several opioid prescriptions to feed their addiction.

Hiding Dependency

Many seniors suffer from forgetfulness that leads them to obtain additional pain medication even though they have a sufficient supply at home. Some simply forget they took their medication earlier in the day and unintentionally double dip. The children, grandchildren, friends and caretakers of the elderly don't detect the opioid addiction. This is primarily due to the fact that the signs of addiction resemble the signs of the aging process. The elderly tend to be forgetful, idle, depressed and irritable.

Some seniors go to great lengths to hide their addiction by taking the extra opioids when no one else is around. If one were to accuse the senior of being addicted to opioids, there is a good chance the senior would passionately deny any dependency. This denial is partially fueled by the addiction itself combined with feelings of guilt. Nobody wants to be a drug addict. Seniors desire to preserve an air of authority and responsibility, especially around family members. As a result, most seniors saddled by opioid addiction tend to feel ashamed by their dependency.

Shame and Denial

The society-wide perception of drug addiction is that it is inherently bad. Society tends to shame those who are hooked on drugs. This negative perception of addicts forces many seniors to deny that they have a dependency. Even family members, friends and caretakers of addicts will deny that there is a problem due to the shame associated with the negative perception of addiction.

Denial is the worst thing that can happen. The addict's problem must be addressed head-on to make progress to a life without a crippling dependency. Family members should not hesitate to interfere with the autonomy of the addicted senior. The truth is, opioid addicts desperately need help. If family members are reluctant to provide assistance

Seniors may go to great lengths to hide their addiction. Denial is the worst thing that can happen.

because they fear a backlash from a fervently independent senior, they will inevitably let the addiction spiral out of control.

An elderly individual's body responds differently to opioids than that of a teen or young adult. The human body becomes more vulnerable as it ages. Bones weaken and muscle mass decreases from the middle of one's life toward the golden years and beyond. If a senior survives an opioid overdose, the fragile body might not be capable of a full recovery. Seniors loaded up on opioids can suffer a nasty fall or misstep that creates irreparable harm. Such an accident can lead to egregiously expensive visits to the emergency room and disability.

Another problem is posed in the form of withdrawal. Seniors who attempt to significantly reduce their opioid intake or go "cold turkey" typically experience severe withdrawal symptoms that trigger relapses. Such relapses are the senior's attempt to prevent even further suffering. Therefore, they should not be shamed for relapsing. These sufferers need compassion and care rather than punishment.

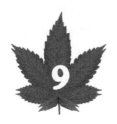

Reducing Opioid Dependency

Studies show cannabis can help with the opioid use explosion in a number of ways. One such study, published in the *Journal of Psychoactive Drugs*, concluded marijuana use can both substitute for opioids and when not completely replacing them, can enhance their effectiveness in ways that will limit their use. When cannabis was used in conjunction with prescription pain medications, fewer pills were needed to achieve the same level of pain relief, thus reducing side effects and limiting tolerance build-up and addiction.

Cannabis is an excellent alternative to painkillers. Cannabis has few side effects compared to powerful pharmaceutical drugs. There is no sense in letting addicts struggle with the

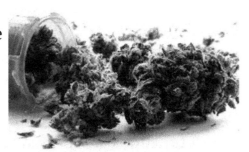

Cannabis has few side effects compared to powerful pharmaceuticals.

intense cravings for painkillers and the incredibly painful physical and mental side effects of these drugs when they can transition to cannabis. Some will even testify that cannabis has helped in their quest to completely cease the use of painkillers.

A University of Michigan study found that those who use cannabis therapy for chronic pain enjoyed a 64 percent decrease in their use of prescription opioid pain medications. These individuals reported that they suffered less side effects from their opioids when used in combination with cannabis. All-in-all, the study's participants reported a 45 percent boost in quality of life after making use of cannabis therapy for pain management. Another cannabis therapy study conducted in Israel across a six month period showed that participants enjoyed a 44 percent reduction in opioid use.

Overdose Not Likely

Another major benefit of cannabis, particularly for seniors, is that while seniors can consume too much cannabis, especially with edibles, and will feel uncomfortable—even miserable—for a few hours, they are not likely to die of an overdose of cannabis. Opioid receptors in the brain are located in the same part of the brain where respiratory functions are located. Cannabinoid receptors, however, are not. This is thought to be why there's never been a recorded overdose fatality from cannabis.

Massachusetts is a hotbed for cannabis therapy. Massachusetts residents who are hooked on opioids were treated with cannabis therapy in a study conducted by the Massachusetts' Canna Care Clinic. The goal of the therapy was to wean the subjects off of highly addictive opioids in favor of non-addictive cannabis therapy. In one study they treated 80 individuals who were hooked on opioids. These addicts progressed through a one-month cannabis therapy program. Over three-quarters of the program's

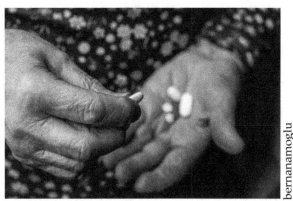

Cannabis can help wean seniors off of highly addictive opioids.

participants ceased use of opioids—an incredible success rate.

Cannabis helps opioid addicts abstain from excessive painkiller use. As a result, these patients enjoy a higher tolerance for opioids. This is due to the fact that cannabis is used as a pain management substitute so the patient does not have to constantly resort to popping pain pills. When a cannabis patients decide to take opioids, they make a much more powerful impact as their tolerance has decreased. As a result, there is less inclination to regain a dependency on opioids.

Withdrawal

Cannabis therapy is especially important for individuals struggling with opioid withdrawal. In fact, some cannabis users report that cannabis use *prevents* opiate withdrawal from occurring in the first place. Cannabis therapy has enabled countless opioid addicts to revert back to the original dose prescribed by the doctor or even a lower dose.

As each day passes, more health leaders ask the medical community to reduce the number of prescription drugs doled out to those in pain. If opioid patients were completely honest, many would testify that they are saddled with a crippling dependency. It is clear that an opioid epidemic is occurring in the United States. It is also clear that cannabis therapy is an excellent alternative to opioids.

Using marijuana can also help mitigate the sometimes very uncomfortable and overpowering side effects of an array of prescription drugs, not to mention the general unpleasantness associated with illness or chronic pain.

> *Cannabis therapy has enabled countless opioid addicts to revert back to the original dose prescribed by the doctor or even a lower dose.*

Not Addictive

Cannabis is not considered to be addictive. Furthermore, the side effects of cannabis pale in comparison to those of opioids. Those who have fallen victim to opioid dependency may find that adding cannabis to be an effective alternative for managing pain. It can reduce the allure of opioids, lower tolerance to opioids and return life to normalcy.

There is a mounting consensus from evidence showing cannabis therapy availability is cutting into opioid use. One such piece of evidence is a study in the *Health Affairs Journal*, which claimed a $165 million reduction in annual Medicare spending on drugs for which marijuana could be a substitute from legalized medical cannabis. Or the *JAMA Internal Medicine* published study that saw a 25 percent reduction in overdoses from painkillers in states with legalized marijuana.

Shifting to Cannabis

People considering using cannabis as a supplement or substitute for opioids or other painkillers should always consult their medical professional. Some doctors endorse the use of cannabis for medical purposes while others still do not. But discussion with a physician is always a must, and can help you to make an informed decision about implementing cannabis products in a prescription regimen.

First time and non-regular users should start slow. When smoking or vaping cannabis in flower (bud) form, one puff should be followed by several minutes of waiting to see how it affects you. The effects can be quick, or sometimes take some time to manifest. One can usually expect a sense of being hungry—commonly called the "munchies", a release of stress, giggling, and deep focus.

As previously mentioned, death from overdose is not a possibility with use of cannabis, so medical attention is only necessary in the case of cardiovascular issues, anxiety or mental health needs, or in some very rare cases, allergic reaction. Fortunately, the majority of cannabis allergies are expressed as nothing more than watery eyes and runny noses, so if you're not feeling well after ingesting or inhaling marijuana, the best cure may just be lying down and relaxing. Certainly one should never operate heavy machinery or drive while under the influence of marijuana, just like one shouldn't while using opioids.

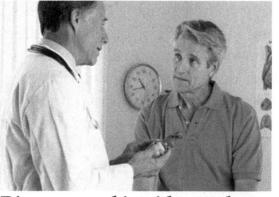
Rocket Clips

With edibles always read the dosage recommendations and instructions very carefully.

Discuss cannabis with your doctor Regardless of

what the packaging says, *always start with a small amount* such as ½ cookie and wait at least an hour for onset of effects before ingesting any more. In fact, it is best to *not* ingest more during the first few uses. Instead, follow the guidelines in Chapter 7: Tailor Your Therapeutics on establishing your baseline and then studying the effects you experience. Then, perhaps the next day or evening, try a small amount more, if effects from the previous session were too subtle—or a little less if the previous results were too strong.

Only you can know if cannabis will be a good substitute or supplement for your existing pain medication. One thing we know is that opioid use can be dangerous and destructive, and while powerful medications can have powerful benefits, particularly for seniors with extreme chronic pain problems, they also come with powerful side effects and risks. Perhaps the best news about trying cannabis is that there is factually very little risk, unlike with prescription narcotics.

Medical science will continue to extend the lives of human beings, and living to older ages, and living with chronic pain for longer will become one of the most important frontiers of medicine. Cannabis is at the forefront of the exploration of that frontier, and might unlock vitality deeper into aging than we've ever known before.

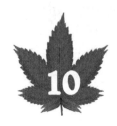

10

Cannabis and Depression

While our lives have vastly improved in the past century, people report feeling less happy than in previous generations, according to Gregg Easterbrook, author of *The Progress Paradox: How Life Gets Better While People Feel Worse*. Depression is a growing problem, especially among seniors.

What is Depression?

Depression is the consistent feeling of sadness and/or a loss of interest. Many depressed people are no longer passionate about once-loved hobbies, work projects, relationships, possessions. Major depression can lead to the complete withdrawal from social activities, physical illness, homelessness and even suicide.

Depression can be induced by social stresses, like job loss. Others endure depression due to psychological stress, like feeling hopeless. Some suffer from depression as a result of biological sources.

Depression is the leading cause of disability in the United States, and worldwide it accounts for more of the disease burden than

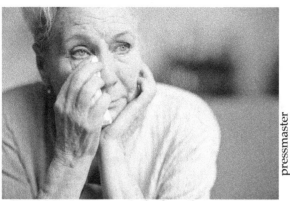

Seniors are at risk for depression.

any other illness but heart disease. Depression can exacerbate social conflicts, abuse, genetics, serious illness, addiction to drugs or alcohol, major life events, social isolation, and even the use of certain medications.

Symptoms

Everybody gets discouraged sometimes. But, if there's a dark cloud hanging over you that persists for weeks or interferes with your ability to function, it may be a case of clinical depression. According to the National Institute of Mental Health, 17 percent of all adults are affected by clinically diagnosed depression which is a serious mental illness.

SYMPTOMS OF DEPRESSION

- *Pessimistic thoughts*
- *Feeling useless and helpless*
- *Chronic unhappiness*
- *No interest in hobbies*
- *Feelings of anxiety or grumpiness*
- *Changes of sleep patterns*
- *Changes in eating habits*
- *Thoughts of Suicide*

When a person has been experiencing symptoms for over two weeks, but does not fill all the same criteria as major depression, this is called "Minor Depression".

"Major Depression" is characterized by an inability to function normally. It can impact schooling, work, leisure, sleeping and eating. This type of depression may only be experienced once but multiple episodes are not uncommon.

Persistent mild depression is called "Dysthymia" and considered chronic. When depression, while mild, lasts for years, it can significantly interfere with relationships and daily activities.

Depression Among Seniors

Seniors tend to suffer from depression at a disproportionately high rate. The elderly are especially prone to depression as the deterioration in physical health accompanying aging can induce feelings of powerlessness and sadness. Older individuals may struggle with exorbitantly high healthcare costs, widowhood, boredom, a lack of purpose, and physical pain. Add in that seniors tend to be isolated and regularly lose friends to death and it is easy to see why seniors suffer from depression at a high rate. Yet depression among seniors tends to be overlooked as the symptoms often resemble those induced by illness and life events expected in the "golden years".

Depression has the potential to cause the deterioration of physical health, drug or alcohol addiction, unemployment/poor work performance, the development of an eating disorder, disconnection from social groups and suicide.

Chronic depression impacts those suffering as well as those around

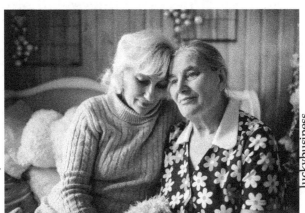

luckybusiness

Loved ones suffer, too.

them. The effects of depression have the potential
to be devastating to the sufferer's loved ones and
friends, as well. It is painful to watch a family
member or friend struggle with depression. Some
loved ones become depressed as a result of a family member's depression. Others sacrifice massive
amounts of time, energy and money attempting
to help the sufferer recover only to make little-to-
no progress.

Treatments

One of the most popular ways to treat depression
is the use of antidepressant medications such as
Prozac, Lexapro, Zoloft, and others. These medications release "happy chemicals" like endorphins and serotonin within the patient's brain.

If you were to poll those who suffer from
depression and rely on antidepressants, many
would claim that the medication really does make
a positive difference. However, there are numerous side effects to these medications ranging from
nausea to constipation, dry mouth, insomnia,
blurred vision, sexual problems, drowsiness and
weight gain.

Talk therapy is another popular treatment for
depression. Seniors who engage in talk therapy
meet with a mental health counselor on a regular
basis. The two engage in discussions where the
senior explains thoughts and feelings in-depth.

The coun-
selor offers
helpful
feedback to
encourages
the patient
to stay ac-
tive, think
positive,
establish
social con-
nections and live a healthy life.

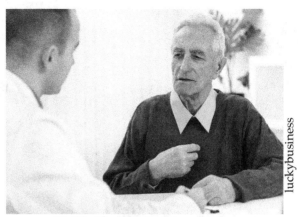

Talk therapy may help.

luckybusiness

This form of treatment is effective for some and ineffective for others. In terms of drawbacks, talk therapy is slow and can be expensive unless the senior has a health insurance plan that provides coverage for mental health services. Talk therapy is quite time-consuming and requires considerable effort on behalf of the senior as well as the therapist.

Alterations to diet and exercise have the potential to improve mood as well as physical well-being. Research shows that a healthy diet combined with regular exercise can ward off depression or mitigate its intensity. Exercise provides a natural high as it releases the aforementioned "happy chemicals" within the senior's brain. Healthy eating combined with exercise over an extended period of time boosts physical attractiveness, which may mitigates feelings of depression.

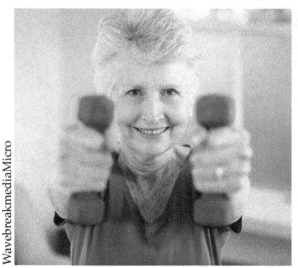

Wavebreakmedia Micro

Exercise releases endorphins that counter depression.

The difficulty with this approach is that few can adhere to a diet and exercise regimen across posterity. This treatment method is especially challenging for those who lack energy as well as those who are entrenched in poor eating habits. Furthermore, improving one's diet and exercise does not address the actual cause of the depression. The true source of the depression must be addressed in order for real change to occur.

Cannabis Can Help

Many are turning to cannabis for relief from depression because it enhances mood and well-being. In fact, cannabis was used as early as the 17th century for depression treatment when Indian doctors doled out the plant to their depressed patients.

Cannabis stimulates the body's endocannabinoid system, hastens the development of nervous tissue, boosts energy, improves focus and decreases anxiety. A plus of cannabis as a treatment modality is that it works relatively quickly, has few (if any) side effects and is inexpensive. Cannabis works faster than antidepressant medications. Though some people experience side effects, like increased appetite or drowsiness, most seniors who try cannabis for depression experience some relief.

Studies conducted at Montreal's McGill University show that low doses of THC generate the "happy chemical" known as serotonin within the patient's brain. Researchers at the Netherlands' University Medical Center Utrecht found that the consumption of THC and CBD activate the brain's endocannabinoid system, prompting the patient to respond in a positive manner to all sorts of stimuli.

Endocannabinoids are chemical compounds produced within the brain. They activate the same receptors as cannabinoids found in the cannabis plant like THC and CBD. When stress is present, the production of endocannabinoids decreases. The result is hindered cognition, negative emotional responses and destructive behaviors. Reduced endocannabinoid production also leads to feelings of anxiety, pain and a deterioration of well-being. Cannabis assists in the production of vitally important endocannabinoids, which consequently, reduces depression.

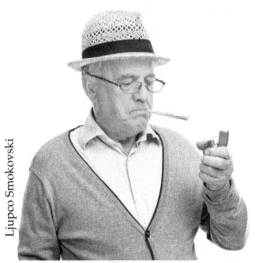

Ljupco Smokovski

Cannabis is especially helpful for those who have anti-social tendencies. Oftentimes, depression causes one to withdraw from social circles and social functions. Many depressed individuals lose interest in relationships, hobbies and social

A few "hits" enlivens mood.

events. Seniors who use cannabis tend to look forward to social interactions as they feel more relaxed and confident. The ensuing social interactions improve mood, self-perception and general well-being.

Using Cannabis to Ease Depression

Some seniors elect to smoke a small amount of cannabis several times a day to improve their mood, calm their nerves and reduce the effects of depression. Depression sufferers should know that several different strains of cannabis are available. Many prefer *sativas*, which boosts energy levels. Many use sativa strains during the morning and afternoon as a "pick me up" to help stay active and productive. Then they turn to *indica* strains in the evening as indicas relax the body and mind. Many also rely on indica strains to enjoy a peaceful night of rest. *Hybrid strains* are an excellent choice for those looking for the best of both worlds.

Inhaling a little cannabis smoke or vapor every few hours can provide rapid relief, helping one make it through the challenges of the day without succumbing to fear, self-doubt and nervousness. It must be noted that especially strong cannabis strains have the potential to worsen depression due to their extremely high THC content. This can be counteracted with cannabidiol (CBD) that provides extensive benefits without the side effects (drowsiness) sometimes caused by THC.

Edibles can be helpful. Eating a low dose cookie or brownie made with cannabis is itself pleasurable. While taking one to two hours for the soothing effects to "come on", the soothing effects last several hours.

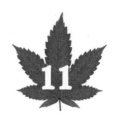

11

Cannabis and Anxiety

Forty million American adults suffer from anxiety-related disorders. A certain amount of anxiety can be a tool to help identify and avert potential threats. It can also motivate us. But out of control anxiety can negatively impact work and relationships. Big Pharma has drugs to reduce anxiety, from selective serotonin reuptake inhibitors (SSRIs) like Prozac and Zoloft, to tranquilizers—the most popular class being benzodiazepines like Valium and Xanax. Many seniors have experienced negative side effects when using such pharmaceuticals.

Described as the sensation of fear and/or panic, anxiety may make

dplett

Anxiety can cripple a senior's life.

people feel nervous and fearful about certain life situations like relationships, job responsibilities, money, school, and so-on. In certain sufferers, feelings of anxiety extend long beyond the end of the situation that induced the fear or nervousness. When anxiety affects a senior's ability to perform everyday functions and enjoy mental clarity, it is a major problem.

The causes of anxiety differ by individual. Anxiety disorders are often induced by a combination of variables such as environmental stress, alterations in the brain, genetics, changes in relationships, substance abuse, and so forth. In many instances, anxiety is a response to external events such as trauma of the death of a loved one, abuse, or stress stemming from relationships, work, finances, illness, school and even the weather. Side effects of medication, exposure to high altitude, anemia, asthma and certain heart conditions can cause anxiety.

Symptoms

Anxiety symptoms range from feeling scared, to feeling panicky and nervous on a consistent basis. Anxiety can be accompanied by feeling depressed, struggling with concentration, difficulties with eating and sleeping, feeling irritable and lacking energy.

Chronic anxiety affects the mind as well as the body. Those who are afflicted may endure health

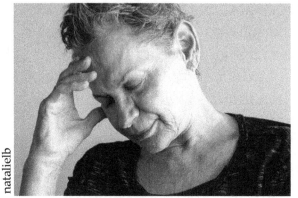

natalielb

problems such as heart palpitations, faintness, diarrhea, dry mouth, trembling, stomach cramps, gastrointestinal disorders, respiratory disorders, heart disease, dizziness, difficulty, swallowing, muscle aches, nausea, shortness of breath, twitching, sweating, or premature coronary artery disease.

Seniors do not have to be plagued by anxiety

Research indicates twice as many seniors are plagued by anxiety than as by depression. The most common mental disorder endured by seniors is generalized anxiety disorder (GAD). Upwards of 14 percent of older adults suffer from some sort of diagnosable anxiety disorder, with about 7 percent of seniors suffering from GAD. According to the *International Journal of Geriatric Psychiatry*, over 27 percent of older adults cared for by a service provider display the symptoms of anxiety.

Though many believe anxiety is a natural part of the aging process, the truth is that seniors do *not* have to be plagued by nervousness and fear. Anxiety makes life difficult for seniors who are supposed to be enjoying their golden years. Oftentimes, seniors face a social void after retiring. For some seniors demands of a stressful career may have prevented them from developing hobbies and relationships so that after retirement they have little to do but remain idle worrying While some worry is normal, excessive worrying for months or years on end is not healthy. For many seniors, this constant state of worry leads to depression, phobias and other psychological distress.

Increases Health Risks

Seniors who suffer from anxiety are at a heightened risk for health problems. Anxious seniors often suffer panic attacks, isolation from others, and social anxiety. Research shows that those who lack a strong social support group tend to be less healthy and die before their socially plugged in peers. Some seniors are so anxious that they do not feel comfortable asking for help from caretakers, family or friends.

Those who suffer from anxiety, or have a loved-one with anxiety, can find comfort in know-

> *Seniors who lack a strong social support group tend to be less healthy and die before their socially plugged in peers.*

ing that there are multiple options for treating anxiety. Prescription medicating, with an array of possible side effects, is no longer the only option for treating anxiety. Cannabis is gaining acceptance amongst medical professionals, politicians and others as a legitimate—and effective—means of reducing anxiety symptoms.

Endocannabinoid System and Anxiety

The body's endocannabinoid system is central to one's ability to regulate anxiety. The body's inherent cannabinoid receptors are abundant in sections of the brain like the hypothalamus and amygdala that are responsible for feelings of anxiety. Studies indicate that the blockage of the body's cannabinoid receptors induce high levels of anxiety. Research also shows that the endocannabinoid system serves to eliminate bad memories and spur the growth of new brain cells. The result of these functions is a decrease in anxiety.

Biphasic Effect

Early research conducted on cannabis's ability to reduce anxiety suggests that the plant might actually trigger long-term anxiety. More recent research indicates that there is a complex relationship between cannabis use and anxiety.

Cannabis compounds have "biphasic properties", which means that low and high doses of the same substance can produce opposite effects. Small doses of cannabis tend to stimulate; large doses sedate. Too much THC, while not lethal, can amplify anxiety and mood disorders. CBD has no known adverse side effects at any dose, but drug interactions can be problematic. An excessive amount of CBD could be less effective therapeutically than a moderate dose. "Less is more" is often the case with respect to cannabis therapeutics.

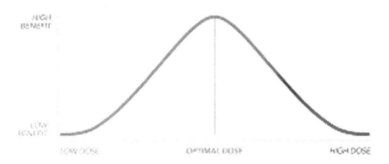

Cannabis compounds have biphasic properties.

The bottom line is the extent to which THC interacts with the neurotransmitter anandamide to make one feel relaxed and happy differs according to each unique senior. Anadamide's effects are mediated primarily by CB1 cannabinoid receptors in the central nervous system, and CB2 cannabinoid receptors in the periphery. The latter are mainly involved in functions of the immune system.

Cannabinoids Help Soothe Anxiety

Many within the medical research community have criticized the above referenced studies as they strictly pertain to pure THC. They argue that the true effects of cannabis on anxiety can only be determined by studying how differing cannabinoid compounds found in marijuana impact anxiety. In particular, the compound known as cannabidiol (CBD) is revered for its ability to decrease anxiety.

Clinical studies and growing evidence from clinical, and epidemiological studies suggest that CBD has powerful anti-anxiety properties. It appears safe, well-tolerated, and may be beneficial to treat a number of anxiety-related disorders.

How Does CBD Work?

CBD exerts several actions in the brain that explain why it could be effective in treating anxiety. Similar to SSRIs, CBD may boost signaling through serotonin receptors. Spanish researchers found that CBD enhances 5-HT1A transmission and may affect serotonin faster than SSRIs. They noted: "The fast onset of antidepressant action of CBD and the simultaneous anxiolytic (anti-anxiety) effect would solve some of the main limitations of current antidepressant therapies."

Brazilian researchers conducted a study of patients afflicted with generalized social anxiety. After consuming CBD, subjects reported a significant decrease in anxiety. When researchers performed brain scans they found that cerebral blood flow patterns were consistent with an anti-anxiety effect.

Other researchers had patients suffering from Social Anxiety Disorder perform a public speaking test. Researchers found that subjects taking CBD showed significantly reduced anxiety, cognitive impairment, and discomfort in their speech performance, as compared to the placebo subjects

Dose

For anxiety, depression, spasms, and pediatric seizure disorders, many patients initially find they do best with a moderate dose of a CBD-dominant remedy (a CBD:THC ratio of more than 10:1).

But a low THC remedy, while not intoxicating, is not necessarily the best therapeutic option. A combination of CBD and THC will likely have a greater therapeutic effect for a wider range of conditions than CBD or THC alone. For cancer, neurological disease, and many other ailments, seniors may benefit from a balanced ratio of CBD and THC.

Extensive clinical research has shown that a 1:1 CBD:THC ratio is effective for neuropathic pain. Optimizing therapeutic use of cannabis entails a careful, step-by-step process, whereby you start with small doses of a non-intoxicating CBD-rich remedy, observe the results, and gradually increase the amount of THC.

Anxiety sufferers have an array of cannabis strains to choose from. The strain selected should be determined by your tolerance level as well as sensitivity to cannabis. Try several strains to

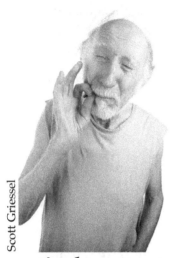

Scott Griessel

A toke or two can soothe anxiety.

determine which is best for your unique anxiety symptoms. Some seniors prefer *indica* strains to put the mind at ease. Alternatively, *sativa* strains tend to energize the body and mind. Experiment with an indica strain to see if it induces a peaceful mindset and relieves stress. Start out with a strain that has a low level of THC and gradually work up to more potent strains if desired.

Some studies show that extensive cannabis use has the potential to create effects similar to those experienced by schizophrenics. If you have a history of mental health issues, do not assume that the regular consumption of cannabis will alleviate your anxiety and produce a perfectly settled mind.

Discuss using cannabis with your health care professional. Cannabis might help certain anxiety sufferers and exaggerate the anxiety of others who are plagued by consistent nervousness and fear. One's mental state, dosage, selected strain, cannabinoid profile and method of ingestion all play a role in determining whether cannabis reduces or worsens anxiety.

Indica

- ⚕ Mainly affects the body
- ⚕ Short and dense plant structure
- ⚕ Heavy feeling and/or "body-melt"

Sativa

- ⚕ Mainly affects the mind
- ⚕ Tall and skinny plant structure
- ⚕ Uplifting and/or euphoric feelings

Start with a strain that is low in THC.

Ideal Method of Ingestion

For those who are extremely anxious and need quick relief, inhalation of cannabis smoke or vapor is rapid acting. Seniors looking for long-term anxiety relief, however, may opt for cannabis edibles or transdermal products like ointments, patches and gels, which can last for many hours at a time. Whatever methods used, always err on the side of using less, especially at first.

Do not assume that the use of cannabis will immediately cure your anxiety. Try different strains to determine which is best for your mind and body. Experiment with different cannabinoid profiles and methods of ingestion before making a final determination as to whether cannabis is the beneficial treatment modality for you.

Cannabis is not a foolproof in treating anxiety. Many anxiety sufferers find significant relief from cannabis. Others who try cannabis find that it makes them feel drowsy or slightly paranoid. Try several cannabis strains to see how they affect your anxiety and follow the process described earlier for developing your personal baseline and evaluating how cannabis works for you.

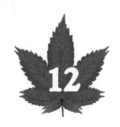

12

Managing Pain

People are living longer, with more vital and active lives, than ever before. Augmented by a constant flow of medical and technological advancements, the human population is thriving and the fastest growing segment of the population is seniors. A study reported in the

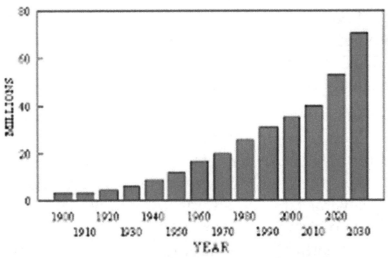

Growth of the Elderly Population
1900 to 2030

Source: U.S. Bureau of the Census

Ochsner Journal estimated the world's population of people over 65 years old will more than double from 500 million to 1.3 billion between 2008 and 2040. With this increase in life expectancy comes an unfortunate new reality: seniors living with chronic pain.

Seniors are Suffering

According to the National Institute of Health, over 75 percent of seniors in assisted living facilities and 50 percent of seniors living on their own struggle with chronic pain. Traditionally, treating chronic pain has been a medical professional prescribing heavy narcotics, opioids and painkillers. These drugs have masked a growing epidemic while causing as many problems as they solve.

Among the most common of the many causes and forms of chronic pain suffered by seniors are joint pain, back pain, neuropathic—nerve—pain, cancer, depression, bone loss, and recovery from injury. These categories include joint issues like osteoarthritis, neuropathic disorders such as sciatica, spinal stenosis, slipped discs and other painful afflictions.

Pain management may include several methods, such as cold laser, acupuncture, traditional and non-traditional physical therapy, and exercise. However, for seniors many of these methods become less effective, dangerous or impossible.

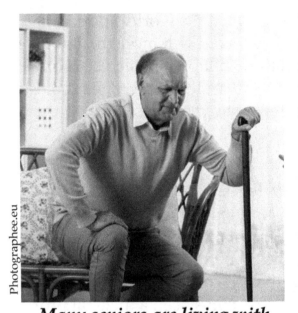

Photographee.eu

Many seniors are living with chronic pain.

The pharmaceutical regimen used to include more reliance on NSAIDs and analgesics, which are non-habit forming. However the threat of side effects, which is magnified in seniors, caused a massive shift toward prescribing strong opioids.

Prescriptions relieve the pain, but do nothing to treat the underlying cause, leading to overreliance, higher tolerance and higher doses of the prescription. It's a vicious cycle that traps vulnerable seniors. Whether living with cancer or arthritis, powerful painkilling prescriptions never actually eliminate the pain.

Compounding the problem is that surgery that might get at the root of the chronic pain, is less attractive to people over 65. The risk of complications, strain on the body, and long recovery times leads many to treat the pain with strong narcotics instead. Similarly, physical therapy that could reduce the source of the pain, as opposed to just masking it, becomes a less tenable option due to the decreased mobility. These factors have created a widespread drug problem in the country, wreaking havoc on seniors.

Failure to adequately treat chronic pain can have tragic consequences. Not infrequently, people in unrelieved pain want to die. Despair can cause patients to discontinue potentially life-saving procedures (e.g., chemotherapy or surgery), which themselves cause severe suffering. In such dire cases, anything that helps to alleviate the pain will prolong and improve these seniors' lives.

Cannabis Soothes Pain

Use of cannabis therapy has been traced back thousands of years. Chinese Emperor Fu Hsi noted the value of cannabis for medicinal purposes in 2900 BCE. In 700 CE, its use for anesthesia and pain relief is documented in the Persian records. In 1611, the British colonial settlers who arrived in Jamestown, Virginia brought marijuana plants with them. The 1621 British tome on mental health, *The Anatomy of Melancholy,*

Prescriptions relieve the pain, but do nothing to treat the underlying cause.

prescribed it as a treatment for depression—both a major side effect *and* cause of chronic pain.

While the numerous ways cannabis can ease chronic pain are yet to be fully understood. What we do know is that it is a viable alternative to opioids and other painkillers, with fewer and less harmful side effects.

Peripheral nerves contain cannabinoid receptors, and the cannabinoids found in cannabis can effectively block those nerves from experiencing pain. An extensive review of studies on cannabis as a pain reliever conducted by the Institute of Medicine found it to be an effective pain reliever for a wide variety of ailments, even rating it on par with the very popular and effective narcotic—codeine. One study found that patients experiencing pain from cancer reported positive pain relief from cannabis therapy, which is notable because chronic pain from cancer shows resistance to opioids.

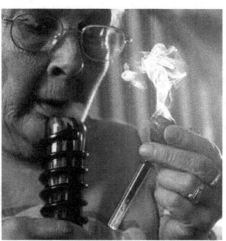

Cannabis affects perception of pain making it easier to ignore.

Several studies have found that cannabinoids have analgesic effects in animal models, sometimes equivalent to codeine. Cannabinoids also seem to synergize with opioids, which often lose their effectiveness as patients build up tolerance. One study found morphine was 15 times more active in rats with the addition of a small dose of THC.

Research from Oxford University showed that unlike opioids or other pain killers, cannabis doesn't seem to activate anything in the part of the brain associated with experiencing pain, rather *it effects one's emotional response to pain.* Said differently, cannabis doesn't numb the pain, rather it affects the *perception* of the pain. That cannabis makes pain bother people less is a huge discovery. It means cannabis therapy can be useful not just as a replacement for traditional

That cannabis makes pain bother people less is a huge discovery.

prescriptions, but as a supplement that can curb overuse, increased dependency and increased tolerance to opioids and other prescriptions. The numbness caused by opioids doesn't just affect the pain, but the senior's concentration, reaction time, ability to think coherently and motor function. The blunting of senses and reflexes can lead to falls and other injuries, an ironic outcome for the use of painkillers.

Nausea

Opioid therapy is often an effective treatment for severe pain, but all opiates have the potential to induce nausea. The intensity and duration of this nausea can cause discomfort and additional suffering that can lead to malnourishment, anorexia, wasting, and a severe decline in a senior's health. Some people find the nausea so intolerable that they are inclined to discontinue the primary pain treatment, rather than endure the nausea. Inhaled cannabis provides almost immediate relief for nausea.

Cannabis can serve two important roles in safe, effective pain management. It can provide relief from the pain itself—either alone or in combination with other analgesics, and it can control the nausea associated with taking opioid drugs, as well as the nausea, vomiting and dizziness that often accompany severe, prolonged pain. In addition, cannabis signifcantly enhances the effectiveness of opioid therapies.

> *Cannabis can provide relief from the pain itself, and it can control the nausea associated with taking opioid drugs.*

Cannabis Relaxes

The accompanying reduction in stress and increase in feelings of relaxation is known to most who have used cannabis. Research shows that relaxation itself promotes healing and pain relief.

Sativa and sativa-dominant hybrid strains generally make one feel more energetic and cerebral.

Because of this, sativas are often preferred for use before exercise and physical therapy. The combination of energetic

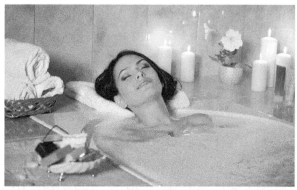

An edible and hot bath and pain floats away.

feeling and focus that comes with sativa often allows patients to work out harder, longer and more effectively, while actually helping in the recovery process.

Indica and indica-dominant hybrid strains are less "active" and deliver less focus and head activity. Indicas are associated with a calming or relaxing effect, which extends to the body—as opposed to the head—causing sensations that can evolve into drowsiness. Indica strains would generally be more effective after physical therapy to aid in relaxing.

Not addictive

Many seniors fear that if they start using marijuana they will become addicted. People can use marijuana daily and then stop "cold turkey". Discontinuing the use of marijuana has much the same response as quitting the consumption of coffee. Many people welcome an effective respite from chronic pain, anxiety, and stress use marijuana as a daily medicine.

Individualize

The best method of use is dependent on the senior, the setting and the ailment. For seniors suffering more acute pain, needing immediate relief, inhalation of combusted flower product or vaporized concentrates will deliver the fastest results, often instantly or within just a few minutes. However, this would likely be a less desirable method of introduction for someone with respiratory or oral distress.

For pain that requires more extended relief, but is less dependent on immediate response, ingestion of edibles or transdermal patches on the skin will be the best method. The effect of the patch or edibles will last much longer, but take longer, often an hour or more, to activate and become apparent.

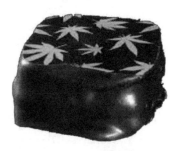

Effects of edibles last a few hours.

Sativas will be more advisable for daytime use for seniors wanting to remain active while using cannabis therapy for pain relief. Indicas, while potentially more potent for pain relief, may cause drowsiness or a lack of desire to be too active, and as such, are more recommended for evening use and before sleep.

Cannabis therapy is changing the lives of chronic pain sufferers. It has many different applications and has different potential benefits. The use of cannabis in pain relief is safer and

> *Cannabis therapy is changing the lives of chronic pain sufferers.*

perhaps more effective than many of the trusted traditional pharmacological methods. The key for seniors is to learn about cannabis therapeutics for pain and to discuss options with their physician. understand the variety and options of cannabis

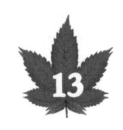

Mind/Body Pain Control

At least 100 million adults in the US suffer from chronic pain, according to the Institute of Medicine. The American Academy of Pain Medicine reports that chronic pain affects more Americans than diabetes, heart disease and cancer combined.

Gate Control Theory of Chronic Pain

Brain researchers describe a kind of nerve gate in the spine that opens to let in certain signals or closes out signals. In times of anxiety or stress, descending messages from the brain may actually amplify the pain signal at the nerve gate as it moves up the spinal cord. Alternatively,

The Gate Control Theory

• The theory states that in the spinal cord there is a neuronal "gate"that signals must pass through. The gate can be open or closed.

•The gate is controlled by movement and other senory information that over-rides pain signals and is specific to the area of pain.

impulses from the brain can "close" the nerve gate, preventing the pain signal from reaching the brain and being experienced as pain.

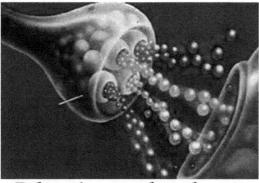

Relaxation can close the gate to pain signals.

When we experience pain, we tend to focus on it and judge its severity, both of which make the pain worse and triggers anxiety. Without meaning to, we amplify pain with our worries about the injury and the pain—and open that nerve gate to more severe pain.

As Johns Hopkins University neuroscience professor David Linden explained, the pain we feel when hurt is controlled and directed by the brain's circuitry. As the brain filters all of the information coming from sensory nerves, it focuses on certain bits and pieces in particular that it might amplify, others that it tones down. Understanding and managing the thoughts, emotions and behaviors that accompany the discomfort can help cope more effectively with pain—and can actually reduce the intensity of "the" pain.

With mind training, in conjunction with the use of cannabis, the nerve gate can be closed to certain pain signals. Training modalities can be roughly divided into sensory—physical being and activities, cognitive—thoughts, and emotions—feelings. Of course in practice there is substantial overlap between these modalities.

Gate Control Theory

The events and conditions that may open the pain gates and cause more suffering include:

Sensory factors, such as injury, inactivity, long-term narcotic use, poor body mechanics, and poor pacing of activities.

Cognitive factors, such as focusing on the chronic pain, having no outside interests or distractions, worrying about the pain, and other negative thoughts.

Emotional factors, such as depression, anger, anxiety, stress, frustration, hopelessness, and helplessness.

Alternatively, influences that can close the pain gates and reduce suffering include:

Sensory factors, such as increasing activities, short-term use of pain medication, relaxation training and meditation.

Cognitive factors, including outside interests, thoughts that help the patient cope with the pain, and distracting oneself from the chronic pain.

Emotional factors, such as having a positive attitude, overcoming depression, feeling reassured that the pain is not harmful, taking control of one's chronic pain and life, and stress management.

Deardorff, William, W., Opening and Closing the Pain Gates for Chronic Pain, *Spine-Health*, March 2003.

Pain is Stressful

Having a painful condition is stressful. Stress can contribute to a range of health problems, including high blood pressure, heart disease, obesity, diabetes, depression and anxiety. Stress can trigger muscle tension or muscle spasms that increases pain. Reducing stress—muscle tension—can affect the intensity of pain experienced.

By learning relaxation techniques, such as deep breathing and meditation, seniors can keep stress levels under control. Stress is an unavoidable part of life, but managing stress helps the body and mind to lessen pain experienced.

Techniques like visualization and mindfulness can help improve quality of life. Dealing with chronic pain is never easy, but when we focus on it less and our spirits lift.

Establish a Pain Baseline

Study your sensation of pain. Where is the pain? How does the pain feel? Is it a burning sensation? Or does it throb? Or tingle? Is it cold? Hot? Are there waves of sensations? Without trying to alter it, dispassionately study the pain. Then rate its intensity or painfulness on a scale from 1 to 9, with 1 being no pain at all and 9 being extreme, nearly unbearable pain.

When first experimenting with using cannabis with mental techniques for soothing pain, it is especially helpful to begin each therapy session by establishing a baseline. Then after the practice, rate your pain level again. In this way, you can detect small improvements, whereas without the baseline it is easy to be overwhelmed that the pain continues and to not notice improvement. Experiencing improvement, namely a soothing and easing of pain, even when small, is success and success is motivating.

Tony Bernhard, author of *How to Live Well With Chronic Pain and Illness* suggests studying a pain-free part of your body. This could be your thumb, your nose, your knee. Study and enjoy the pain-free sensation, allowing it to enlarge.

Bernhard advises that benefit is gained by looking for other pleasant sensations. For example, notice the warmth of the blanket you are laying upon; the feel of the sun streaming through the window; the sound of children laughing outside; a fleeting thought about looking forward to seeing a friend; an odor coming from the kitchen. Focusing upon sensory inputs instead of the pain can help to ease it.

Breathe Deeply

Start by sitting or lying down in a comfortable position. Pay attention for a minute or two to the

physical sen-
sation of your
breath as it
goes in and
out of your
body.

Now
breathe in
while slowly
counting to
three: "One-

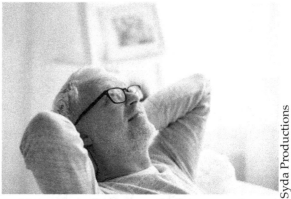

Breathe slowly while counting breaths.

Syda Productions

and-two-and-three". Then hold your breath
for two to three seconds, then slowly breath out
while again counting to three: "One-and-two-
and-three". Doing this simple exercise will relax
your body in a few minutes. Using cannabis,
especially a low dose edible about an hour before
the breathing practice, can greatly deepen the
enperience.

Relax Muscles Directly

After breathing deeply for 3-4 minutes, scan your
body from head to toe to discover muscles that
are tight. Then while focusing on that muscle,
tense the muscle while taking a slow deep breath,
holding the breath and tensed muscle for 2-3 seconds, and then exhale while quickly releasing the
tension from the muscle, and thinking, "Relax".
Repeat this with each tense muscle. Take your
time in doing this. There is no rush.

Visualize Wellness

When visualizing, see or picture in your mind
some action that removes or cures the pain. As
with other mind-body techniques, always begin
by relaxing yourself with deep breathing for 4-5
minutes. Then imagine some action curing or
removing "the" pain. For example suppose your
knee is aching. You might see yourself in a beauti-
ful pool with lush plants and a wonderful water-
fall of special holy water running over your knee
and washing the pain away.

The curative action you imagine does have to
be "logical", it must simply take the pain away
in your vision. You might envision a wizard with
a wand, which taps your knee to make the pain
gone. Or you might picture a large vat of delicious cannabis butter poured over your knee and
dissolving the pain. Using cannabis when visualizing can intensify your imagination for a more
powerful experience.

Distract Yourself

When pain flares, find ways to distract your mind
from it. Watch a movie, take a walk, engage in a
hobby or visit a museum. Pleasant experiences
can help you cope with pain. Using cannabis can
augment your ability to distract yourself from
"the" pain—not "your" pain.

Dissociate From "the" Pain

Imagine that the painful part of your body is separate from the rest of your body, far away from your mind. You might visualize your pain as a giant blob, a loud noise, or a bright light. Then imagine that you are gradually reducing it—shrinking the size of the blob, lowering the noise, or dimming the light. Again, a few tokes of a cannabis joint or vape can amplify the distance between you and "the" pain—over there.

Meditate

Numerous studies have shown that meditation substantially reduces pain and may actually change how the brain processes pain. Done correctly, meditation can help pain suffers move their focus away from their body.

Start with a low dose of cannabis, with brief sessions of 10 to 15 minutes so the practice is not too overwhelming or burdensome. Begin each meditation by counting your breaths as you breathe slowly and deeply to enter the meditative state.

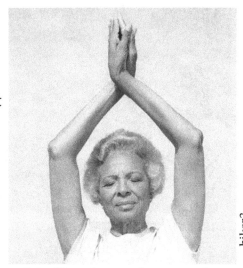

biker3

Meditation reduces pain.

Laugh

Laughter can reduce pain by releasing endorphins. We've all heard of—and may have experienced—pot and the giggles. Smoking a little cannabis encourages an enlivened mood and seeing hassles as indicative of "The Cosmic Chuckle".

So going to a comedy club or seeing your favorite comedy film can, quite literally, be therapeutic—especially when enjoyed with perhaps a cannabis edible eaten an hour or so before the performance.

Enjoy Music

Listening to music is another activity shown to be successful in helping people ease chronic pain. Studies have shown that listening to music as little as one hour a day reduces chronic pain. Music decreases pain and feelings of depression while increasing the listener's sense of power. Studies show that "pleasing" music, in particular, offers the most pain reduction.

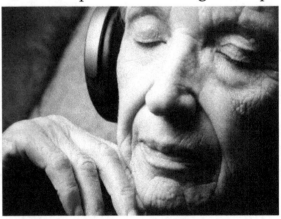

kuzmafoto

Listening to music eases pain and enlivens mood.

Be Social

Seniors suffering chronic pain often withdraw from social activity. But doing so is counterproductive. Making plans with family and friends can boost mood and distract from "the" pain. In fact, simply thinking of friends and family reduces pain. Studies show that viewing pictures of loved ones, such as romantic partners, increases the body's resistance to pain.

Enjoying a few tokes of cannabis while looking at the photos just makes it more enjoyable. A cannabis edible about an hour before meeting up with friend or family can have you feeling convivial and upbeat, full of optimism.

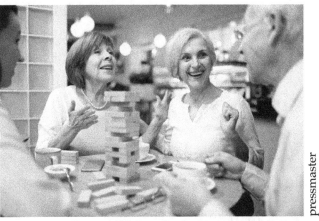

A cannabis edible about an hour before meeting up with friend or family can have you feeling convivial and upbeat, full of optimism.

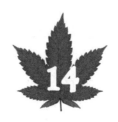

Neuroprotection

Neurodegeneration is an umbrella term for the progressive loss of structure or function of neurons, including death of neurons, found in degenerative nerve diseases, which are serious and can be life-threatening. Most have no cure. With research showing that cannabinoids have neuro-protective powers for healing, there is finally a light at the end of the tunnel.

Neurodegenerative Diseases

Degenerative nerve diseases affect many of the body's activities, such as balance, movement, talking, breathing, and heart function. Seniors living with neurode-generative diseases can endure an insurmountable amount of pain on a daily basis.

Excitotoxicity is the pathological process by which neurons are damaged and killed by the overactivations of receptors for the excitatory neurotransmitter glutamate.

While many of these diseases have genetic roots; more often the cause is a medical condition such as alcoholism, a tumor, or a stroke. Other causes include high levels of oxidative stress, mitochondrial dysfunction, inflammation, various forms of neurotoxicity—e.g. excitotoxicity, protein deficiencies, and viruses. Too often, however, the cause is not known.

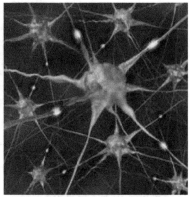

Nerve cells and functioning are damaged.

Stroke

Ischemic stroke is the fifth leading cause of death in the United States and a leading cause of adult disability. When a blood vessel carrying blood to the brain is blocked by a clot or plaque, an ischemic stroke occurs because blood cannot reach the brain, thereby depriving it of oxygen. High blood pressure is the most common risk factor for this type of stroke. Ischemic strokes account for about 87% of all strokes.

Parkinson Disease

Parkinson's disease is characterized by loss of dopamine neurons in the substantia nigra of the

> *The aim of neuroprotection is to slow and preferably halt the loss of neurons.*

brain, affecting about 3 percent of the popula- tion over the age of 65. At the time of clinical diagnosis generally patients have already lost 60 percent or more of the neurons in the substantia nigra pars compacta. Pharmacologic treatment of Parkinson disease is divided into two therapeutic models: neuroprotective and symptomatic therapy. While there is much optimism about neuroprotective therapy and its potential benefits, in practice it is still largely theoretical because most available treatments are symptomatic and do not appear to slow or reverse the natural course of the disease.

Alzheimer's Disease

Alzheimer's is a progressive disease, where dementia symptoms gradually worsen over a number of years. In its early stages, memory loss is mild, with difficulty remembering newly learned information because Alzheimer's changes typically begin in the part of the brain that affects learning. With late-stage Alzheimer's, victims experience personality change, lose the ability to carry on a conversation or to respond to their environment. While the greatest known risk factor is increasing age and the majority of people with Alzheimer's are 65 and older, *Alzheimer's is not a normal part of aging.*

Multiple Sclerosis

Multiple Sclerosis is a long-lasting disease that affects the brain spinal cord, and the optic nerves in the eyes, resulting in problems with vision, balance, muscle control, and other basic body functions.

MS happens when the immune system attacks a fatty material called "myelin" that wraps around nerve

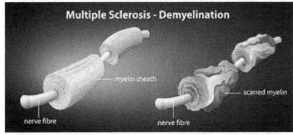

Multiple Sclerosis - Demyelination

myelin sheath

scarred myelin

nerve fibre   *nerve fibre*

The immune system attacks fatty material that wraps around nerve fibers to protect them

fibers to protect them. The resulting scar tissue prevents the brain from sending signals correctly through the body. When immune cells activate, they release pro-inflammatory proteins called "cytokines" that cause rampant inflammation in the brain. This ultimately results in the destruction of neurons, and progressively worsening symptoms.

Amyotrophic Lateral Sclerosis

Amyotrophic lateral sclerosis, also known as Lou Gehrig's disease, is a progressive neurodegenerative disease affecting nerve cells in the brain and the spinal cord. Motor neurons reach from the brain to the spinal cord and from the spinal cord to the muscles throughout the body—all of which degenerate as the disease progresses.

Neuroprotective Agents

Research increasingly suggests that much of the cognitive decline associated with aging can be slowed or mitigated with neuroprotection, a newly studied process believed capable of slowing and—even preventing—nerve damage, thereby preserving some or all cognition and mental performance.

Neuroprotective agents are substances that protect brain function and structure, protecting against nerve cell degeneration. Increasingly research evidence confirms that neuroprotective agents help improve mitochondrial and neurotransmitter function by improving signaling between neurons. Others protect the dopamine neurons and the retina. The majority of neuroprotective agents are antioxidants. There is growing evidence that certain cannabinoids have neuroprotective powers.

There is growing evidence that certain cannabinoids have neuroprotective powers.

Cannabis Neuroprotection

Various cannabinoids have been found in rodent studies to have neuroprotective properties. Particularly THC and cannabidiol CBD have both been shown to reduced levels of NMDA and AMPA induced neurotoxicity, supporting that the cannabinoids have antioxidant benefits and may protect the brain from glutamate-based neurotoxicity.

While performing experiments on cannabis, Sackler Faculty of Medicine researcher Dr. Yosef Sarne discovered that low doses of THC have a significant impact on cell signaling, preventing cell death and promoting growth factors. Sarne's research, published in *Behavioral Brain Research* and *Experimental Brain Research*, demonstrated that extremely low doses of THC administered over a wide window of 1 to 7 days

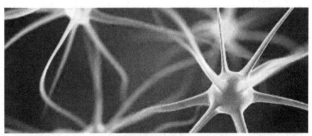

Low doses of THC have a significant impact on cell signaling, preventing cell death and promoting growth factors.

before or 1 to 3 days after injury can jumpstart biochemical processes that protect brain cells and preserve cognitive function over time. Sarne concluded that use of THC may prevent long-term cognitive damage resulting from brain injury.

Stroke

The cannabinoid CBD has been subject of much investigation is a neuroprotectant for strokes. For example, CBD has been shown to increase cerebral blood flow following a stroke, thereby aiding in mitigating infarct volume. While research indicates that THC has similar benefits, CBD is believed to have greater therapeutic potential than THC because it remains effective after fourteen days of repeated treatment, whereas THC tends to decrease in effectiveness with repeated doses. Additionally, CBD has been shown to reduce inflammation caused by release of interleukin-1, nitric oxide, and tumour necrosis factor-a following stroke.

Reactive oxygen species (ROS) are formed as a natural byproduct of the normal metabolism of oxygen and have important roles in cell signaling and homeostasis. During times of environmental stress, such as heat exposure, however, ROS levels can increase dramatically to severely damage to cell structures, known as "oxidative stress."

As with traumatic brain injury, much of the damage following a stroke is due to oxidative stress, which is caused by the build-up of reactive oxygen species (ROS) resulting from the excessive glutamatergic signaling. Both THC and CBD have been shown to be effective antioxidants that inhibit glutamatergic signaling and thereby reduce the extent of ROS build-up following ischemic stroke. Notably, CBD again shows greater effectiveness as an antioxidant than does THC—suggesting its greater therapeutic potential than THC.

Alzheimer's Disease

A study conducted by Dr. Neel Nabar published in the *Journal of Alzheimer's Disease* found that very small doses of THC slows the production of beta-amyloid proteins—thought to be a key contributor to the progression of Alzheimer's. A study from the Salk Institute found that THC and other compounds in cannabis reduce the amount of beta amyloid in the brain. The Salk Senior Researcher, Dr. David Schuber found that exposure to THC reduced the levels of beta amyloid, stopped the inflammatory response from the nerve cells caused by beta amyloid and allowed the nerve cells to survive.

Additional support comes from animal research in which subject mice were injected with a single low dose of THC before exposing them to brain trauma. The control mice also sustained brain injury but did not receive the THC treatment. After five weeks, subject mice treated with THC performed better on behavioral tests measuring learning and memory. Biopsies showed heightened amounts of neuroprotective chemicals in the subject mice as compared to the controls.

Multiple Sclerosis

Research suggests that endocannabinoids can reduce spasticity in multiple sclerosis. Professor of Clinical Neuroscience at University of St. Andrews U.K. Dr. John Zajicek conducted clinical trials on pain and spasticity in multiple sclerosis with results supporting anecdotal reports of symptomatic improvement, particularly for muscle stiffness and spasms, neuropathic pain and sleep and bladder disturbance, in patients with MS treated with cannabinoids. Zajicek reported that experimental evidence suggests that cannabinoids effect more fundamental processes operating in MS, with evidence of anti-inflammation, encouragement of remyelination and neuroprotection. Considered the foremost authority on cannabis and neurodegenerative diseases, Zajicek concluded that evidence for a beneficial effect of cannabinoids on symptomatic spasms and spasticity is persuasive.

In a study conducted by University of California, Dr. Corey-Bloom examined the short-term effect of smoked cannabis on spasticity. Thirty-seven subjects were assigned to smoke cannabis containing 4 percent THC or placebo cigarettes once daily for three days. Findings showed that smoked cannabis reduced pain and treatment-resistant spasticity associated with MS better than the placebo group.

Researcher Dr. G. Pryce found that synthetic cannabidiol can slow accumulation of disability from the inflammatory penumbra during relapsing experimental autoimmune encephalomyelitis in mice, possibly via blockade of voltage-gated sodium channels. Pryce said it is promising that the neurodegeneration that drives progressive disability can be limited.

> *Data showed symptomatic improvement for muscle stiffness and spasms, neuropathic pain and sleep and bladder disturbance, in patients with MS treated with cannabinoids.*

A word of caution: A research team led by Dr. Anthony Feinstein at Sunnybrook Research Institute in Toronto demonstrated that smoked cannabis can negatively affect cognition in people with MS, impeding their ability to perform tasks related to information processing speed, working memory, executive functions, and visuospatial perception. So it is important to determine the potential neuropsychological effects of cannabis use, which may add further difficulty to performing basic tasks and thought processes.

Implications for Seniors

While more research to establish neuroprotection is needed, there is much optimism. Most exciting is the possibility that cannabinoids may be an effective neuroprotective agent with a wide role than symptom alleviation. There is considerable experimental evidence that cannabinoids are associated with reduced excitotoxicity secondary to reduced neurotransmitter release, synaptic modulation, reduced free radical damage, improved mitochondrial function and reduced inflammation along with increased repair and remyelination.

Considering that the downside of using cannabis is minimal, especially when compared to use of powerful pharmaceuticals, seniors should discuss with their physician adding cannabis to their treatment regime. It will reduce inflammation and the accompanying pain as well as mitigating other distressing symptoms.

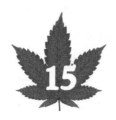

Cannabis and Chemo

Research suggests that THC and other cannabinoids such as CBD can slow the growth and cause death in certain types of cancer cells in laboratory dishes. Some animal studies suggest certain cannabinoids may slow growth and reduce spread of some forms of cancer. Early clinical trials of using cannabinoids to treat cancer in humans have shown that cannabinoids can be safe in treating cancer, but thus far they do not show that they help control or cure the disease.

Relying on marijuana alone as treatment while avoiding or delaying conventional medical care for cancer may have serious health consequences.

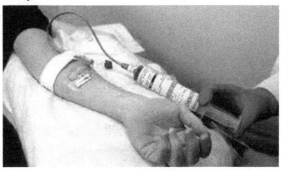

Chemo is a massive assault to the body.

Counter Chemo Side Effects

Chemotherapy is a cancer treatment that uses strong drugs, administered orally or intravenously. These drugs prevent cancer from spreading to other parts of the body, slow the growth of tumors, and kill cancer cells. While chemotherapy can be effective against cancer, it causes serious side effects.

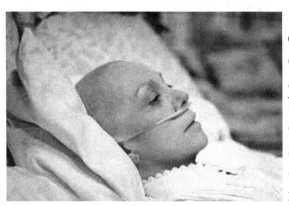

Chemo causes considerable suffering.

The side effects from chemotherapy develop because the chemotherapy drugs damage normal, healthy cells while preventing the cancerous cells from spreading. Side effects associated with chemotherapy include fever and chills, fatigue, nausea and vomiting, sore mouth, diarrhea, constipation, loss of appetite and weight loss, pain or difficulty with swallowing, swelling in the hands or feet, itching, shortness of breath, cough, and muscle or joint pain. The severity of the side effects varies greatly from person to person. Most side effects gradually go away after completion of the treatment.

FDA Approved Cannabis Drugs

Two chemically pure drugs based on cannabis compounds have been approved in the US for medical use.

Dronabinol (Marinol®) is a gelatin capsule containing delta-9-tetrahydrocannabinol (THC) approved by the FDA to treat nausea and vomiting caused by cancer chemotherapy.

Nabilone (Cesamet®) is a synthetic cannabinoid that acts much like THC approved to treat nausea and vomiting caused by cancer chemotherapy.

Nabiximols is a cannabinoid mouth spray drug made up of a whole-plant extract with THC and cannabidiol (CBD) under study to treat pain linked to cancer.

Research has shown that using cannabis can reduce the nausea and vomiting that often occurs after chemotherapy treatments. Researchers Rocha et.al. found that CBD is effective at treating nausea, as well as preventing anticipatory nausea in chemotherapy patients. In another study Limebeer and Parker found that THC is effective at reducing chemotherapy-induced nausea.

Cannabis can help prevent weight loss and a loss of appetite in chemotherapy patients. Nelson et.al. showed that THC can stimulate appetite in patients that have cachexia related to cancer.

Chemotherapy patients treated with THC report increased appetite and that food "tastes better" in a study by Brisbois et.al.

Research by Burstein and Zurier suggests that cannabis can reduce the swelling in the hands and feet that chemotherapy patients often experience. In a study by Bar-Sela et.al. of 131 cancer patients receiving cannabis treatments for six to eight weeks reported significant improvements in nausea, vomiting, mood disorders, fatigue, weight loss, anorexia, constipation, sexual function, sleep disorders, itching, and pain. Brisbois research group found that patients treated with THC have also been shown to experience a higher quality of sleep and relaxation. The National Cancer Institute endorsed cannabis as an effective treatment for providing relief of a number of symptoms associated with cancer and chemotherapy treatments, including pain, nausea and vomiting, anxiety and loss of appetite.

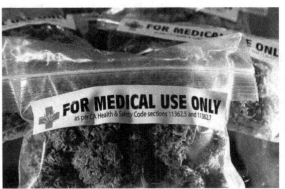

Oncologists are looking to cannabis to manage effects of chemo.

A growing number of cancer patients and oncologists view the cannabis as a viable alternative for managing chemotherapy's effects, as well as some of the physical and emotional health consequences of cancer, such as bone pain, anxiety and depression. A 2014 poll conducted by Medscape and WebMD found that more than three-quarters of American physicians think cannabis provides real therapeutic benefits. 82 percent of oncologists in their study agreed that cannabis should be offered as a treatment option.

Dr. Donald Abrams, chief of hematology-oncology at San Francisco General Hospital and a professor of clinical medicine at the University of California, San Francisco. Marijuana, says cannabis "is the only anti-nausea medicine that increases appetite." It also helps patients sleep and elevates their mood according to Abrams.

Killing Cancer Cells

Cancer cells are covered with cannabinoid receptors. The CB1 cannabinoid receptor on the cancer cell creates a waxy lipid molecule called ceramide

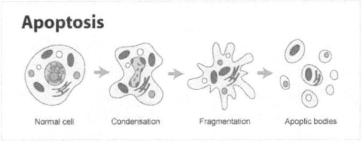

Apoptosis

Normal cell   Condensation   Fragmentation   Apoptic bodies

Apoptosis is programmed cell death.

that disrupts the cell's mitochondria, which prevents the cell from getting energy, causing the
cancer cell to die.

Unlike necrosis, a process called apoptosis is
controlled cell death that doesn't damage surrounding cells. Recent studies found that cannabis may trigger apoptosis in cancer cells. This
exciting development suggests that treatment
focused on a tumor can kill cancer cells while
minimizing risk to healthy cells and tissue.

Work With Your Doctor

When introducing cannabis into your treatment
protocol is it vital to always work with your personal physician. Cannabis can soothe nausea and
relieve the pain associated with cancer but using
cannabis alone to treat cancer would be a mistake.
While there are early indications that cannabis
may slow tumor growth, there are no firm results—yet!

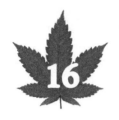

A Good Night's Sleep

The National Institute of Health reports that almost 50 percent of seniors struggle with insomnia, which is the difficulty of falling or staying asleep. "Insomnia is common for seniors, partly because of health issues, partly because of the anxiety and the concerns of aging, and sometimes because of medications," says Dr. Jack Gardner, MD, a neurologist at the Sleep Center at Baylor Medical Center.

Quality sleep is as important as quantity for rejuvenating the body. Many seniors report being less satisfied with sleep and more tired during the day. Lack of sleep has the potential to cause memory loss, headaches, depression, cardiovascular disease, diabetes mellitus, renal failure, respiratory diseases such as asthma, and immune disorders.

Studies on the sleep habits of American seniors show an increase in the time it takes to fall asleep—sleep latency, an overall decline in REM sleep, and an increase in sleep fragmentation—

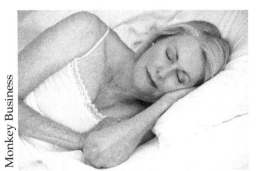

Monkey Business

Quality of sleep is as important as quantity.

waking up during the night—with age. The prevalence of sleep disorders also tends to increase with age. However, research suggests that much of the sleep disturbance among seniors can be attributed to physical and psychiatric illnesses and the medications used to treat them.

Sleep Apnea

Snoring is the primary cause of sleep disruption for approximately 90 million American adults. Snoring is commonly associated with being overweight—a condition often becoming worse with age. Loud snoring is particularly serious as it can be a symptom of obstructive sleep apnea—OSA—and is associated with high blood pressure—putting seniors at risk for cardiovascular disease, headaches, memory loss and depression, according to Dr. Michael Vitiello's research with National Institute on Aging.

With OSA, breathing stops—sometimes for as long as 10-60 seconds—and the amount of oxygen in the blood drops, which alerts the brain, causing a brief arousal or awakening, then breathing resumes. These stoppages of breathing can occur repeatedly, causing multiple sleep disruptions throughout the night, causing excessive daytime sleepiness and impaired daytime function.

Untreated sleep apnea is a serious disorder that is easily treated. Talk to your doctor if you experience snoring on a regular basis, especially if it can be heard from another room or you have been told you stop breathing or make loud or gasping noises during sleep— all symptoms of sleep apnea.

Other Sleep Deprivation Problems

Restless legs syndrome (RLS) is a neurological movement disorder characterized by an irresistible urge to move the limbs. With RLS, unpleasant, tingling, creeping or pulling feelings occur mostly in the legs, becoming worse in the evening, making it difficult to stay asleep during the night. Prevalence increases with age, with about 10 percent of seniors reported to experience RLS symptoms. About 80 percent of people with RLS also have periodic limb movement disorder—PLMD.

Gastroesophageal reflux disease—GERD—is another common cause of sleep problems. The pain of GERD makes sleeping a challenge. Diseases such as Parkinson's disease and multiple sclerosis also commonly cause problems sleeping.

Untreated sleep apnea is a serious disorder that is easily treated.

Sleep Patterns

Changes in sleep patterns are a part of normal aging. Seniors tend to have a harder time falling asleep and more trouble staying asleep than when they were younger. However, it is a common misconception that sleep needs decline with age. Actually, research has demonstrated that sleep needs remain constant throughout adult life.

Changes in the patterns of sleep—called sleep architecture—occur with aging, which may contribute to sleep problems. While drifting off, the body enters into NREM—non-rapid-eye-movement—sleep and goes through four stages, beginning with light sleep, progressing to deeper sleep. During the fifth stage, known as REM—rapid eye movement—sleep, breathing becomes irregular and shallow, eyes move rapidly, limb muscles become immobile, and dreaming may occur. The entire NREM-REM cycle lasts about 90-110 minutes, and usually takes place 4-5 times during normal sleep.

The sleep cycle is repeated several times during the night and although total sleep time tends to remain constant, seniors spend more time in the lighter stages of sleep than in deep sleep.

It is a common misconception that sleep needs decline with age.

Consult Your Doctor

If you're experiencing difficulty getting to sleep and staying asleep always discuss your symptoms with your doctor. It is helpful to keep a record of your sleep and fatigue levels throughout the day and any other symptoms you might take with you when consulting with your doctor.

Your doctor may prescribe a medication to help you sleep. The particular medication prescribed to treat insomnia depends on your diagnosis, medical condition, use of alcohol or other drugs, age, and need to

> *Sleep medications can lead to tolerance, withdrawal symptoms, and rebound insomnia.*

function when awakened during the usual sleep period. Sleep medications can lead to tolerance, withdrawal symptoms, and rebound insomnia. Pharmaceutical medication should be used only as recommended by your doctor. Never use drugs given by a friend or relative. If you are interested in trying cannabis as a sleep aid, make sure to discuss it with your doctor before you stop using medication prescribed to help you sleep.

Cannabis As Sleep Aid

Many seniors find using cannabis is helpful with treating sleep issues. In many instances, cannabis therapeutic alleviates these ailments, making it a restful night of sleep possible.

As an example, cannabis therapy improves breathing during sleep, which is vitally important for seniors suffering from sleep apnea and endure regular obstructions of breath causing them to wake several times during the night, and to endure health problems like mood disturbances, fatigue, inattention, daytime sleepiness, headaches and a greater chance of being involved

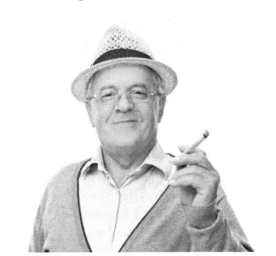

Ljupco Smokovski

In-taking a small amount of THC helps individuals get to sleep quickly.

in some kind of accident, including while driving.

Preclinical studies indicate using cannabis helps reduce sleep apnea. One study showed that THC restores respiratory stability with the modulation of serotonin signaling. This is quite helpful for sleep apnea patients. Another study performed showed that the exogenous cannabinoid called dronabinol—Marinol—is helpful for sleep apnea sufferers enabling them to enjoy a continuous night's sleep.

How Cannabis Helps

Using cannabis promotes restful sleep in a number of ways. Research suggests that in-taking a small amount of THC helps individuals get to sleep quickly. Cannabis is believed to hasten the transition from stage one sleep to stage two, which enables one to get to sleep without delay, as well as reducing tossing and turning during the night to enjoy a solid night of sleep and wake feeling refreshed.

Dreams occur during the final stage of the sleep cycle called REM sleep. using cannabis lengthens the amount of time spent in the third stage of sleep, which is the restorative sleep stage. Since this stage is lengthened, scientists believe that the reduced REM sleep caused by cannabis therapy might not be significant.

Because dosing of THC may be tricky, using cannabis sativa within a few hours before bedtime should probably be avoided. The use of cannabis indica strains is recommended for sleep enhancement. Indica calms the body and mind, allowing one to obtain a restful sleep. This is a striking contrast to sativa cannabis strains that kick-start the body and mind sort of like a cup of coffee.

DNA and chemical testing research has not shown how indicas improve sleep. Many believe the terpene content is responsible. Terpenes are the aromatic compounds that partially make up each cannabis strain's unique fingerprint. It is believed that indica cannabis strains have an abundance of the relaxing terpenes as compared to sativa strains.

Cannabinol—CBN—is the cannabinoid scientists point to as the source of cannabis' sedative effects. CBN stems from cannabigerolic acid—CBGA—in cannabis. The plant naturally produces enzymes through the synthases process that converts the CBGA to one of 3 major cannabinoids: cannabichromene carboxylic acid—CBCA, cannabidiol carboxylic acid—CBDA, and tetrahydrocannabinol carboxylic acid—THCA.

Another study showed the effects of cannabis with high CBD provides therapeutic help for daytime sleepiness due to the inability to sleep soundly at night. This condition is called somnolence.

Age of cannabis is another factor. Aged cannabis tends to promote better sleep than young cannabis. As THC degrades across time, it transforms into the sedating chemical of CBN. Aged cannabis with high CBN is upwards of five times as sedating as THC.

Consider Edibles

All of this is rather confusing and may point to experimenting with low dose edibles to improve sleep. Edibles can be obtained at a cannabis dispensary or you may experiment with making your own.

In either case, 1) start with a low dose, and 2) avoid sugar. Remember that effects "come on" slowly with

Your sleep will not be helped if you eat too much edible and you have a bad reaction.

edibles, generally about an hour, because the cannabis-laced food must go through the digestion system and into the intestines to finally enter the blood where it gets carried through out the body. Your sleep will not be helped if you eat too much and suffer a bad reaction and you may then be fearful of trying edibles again. Start small. Use the data collecting method described earlier to study your insomnia and then to study the subtle affects of small dose edibles.

Secondly, avoid sugar. Not only is sugar a stimulant, that is likely to awaken rather than subdue you, but it is related to many horrific conditions like, most especially, to cancer. If you can't find low-sugar edibles where you shop, you may need to makes your own.

Ask those who have taken sleeping medication and there is a good chance they will testify to feelings of grogginess when waking. This is not the case with cannabis therapeutics. The use of cannabis promotes a lengthy and replenishing sleep that allows seniors to feel energized upon waking. This is the type of refreshing and energizing sleep everyone deserves.

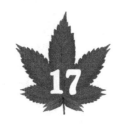

Quelling Discomforts

Using cannabis can have discomforting side effects for some seniors new to cannabis. Generally these discomforts result from an overactive imagination and can be avoided through relaxation, distraction and positive thinking. Here are ways to resolve such discomforts for seniors new to using cannabis and its properties.

Fear and Worry

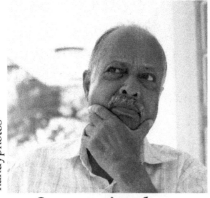

Some seniors have trepidation about using cannabis.

Some seniors have trepidation when they first use cannabis because it is such a unique experience. In this case, seniors can prepare by relaxing and reminding themselves that they are fine and in control of the situation.

A comprehensive study that explored how cannabis can cause short-term paranoia was lead by Oxford Professor Daniel Freeman and funded by the Medical Research Council. Scientists observed 121 individuals between the ages of 21 and 50. Participants had no history of mental problems and had used cannabis in the past. Two thirds of the subjects were injected with THC, another third was given a placebo. The THC had the impact of a 90 minute high. Half of the THC subjects said they had suspicious fearful thoughts, whereas only 30 percent of the placebo participants reported paranoid thinking. As THC exited the bloodstream of its users, the paranoia decreased as well.

Freeman concluded that low self-esteem and worry combined with cannabis could lead to paranoid thoughts in some individuals. He defined paranoia as "excessive thinking that other people are trying to harm us." Even though THC seemed to provide a cause and effect relationship regarding paranoia, the researchers concluded that paranoia can be triggered by multiple causes. They did not link their study to long-term effects.

Freeman suggested that the individuals focus on self-confidence and avoid worrying about who might cause them harm. He noted that the effects of THC as it interacts with the endocannabinoid system are directly related to dosage, so those who experience uncomfortable para-

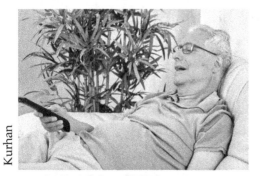

Kurhan

Watching TV is a great distraction.

noia may opt for a lower dosage or move on to a more comfortable strain. CBD can also be used as a gate-keeper that regu-lates how much THC interacts with receptors.

It also helps to use games as a distraction to take the mind off worries. Engaging in laughter by watching a comedy show or joking with friends diminishes the doom and gloom feelings of paranoia. Keeping the mind active is part of the solution. Being physically active is also helpful. Serotonin, which maintains mood balance is released when exercising. Finally, naps can help sleep off discomfort.

Dizziness

Cannabis may cause a dizzy sensation known as vertigo in some individuals. It's been described as similar to the awkward rush some people feel after riding on a rollercoaster. The exact reason cannabis causes dizziness has yet to be confirmed by scientists, although the main culprit appears to be THC.

One theory is that THC can modify sensory perception, leading to disorientation. Such disorientation can trigger anxiety, which can speed up heart rate and weaken neurological processes.

Part of overcoming dizziness is to minimize the chances of potential accidents, such as falling down. While severe dizziness is not typical, but if dizziness lasts longer than a few hours, it may require medical help. Standing up slowly helps dizzy seniors maintain balance. If one ever feels they lack balance standing up, they should sit down and breathe slowly to relax.

Seniors who have experienced dizziness should use smaller doses and pay close attention to potency. They should remind themselves that the high is temporary. Avoiding fast motion can help reduce dizziness; taking deep breaths and releasing air slowly may help eliminate dizziness, as well.

Memory Loss

"Stoners" have always been tagged as forgetful, such as misplacing keys, pens or phones. The euphoric effect of cannabis can create a "spaced out" sensation, in which the brain delivers information at a slower pace, leading to obvious details getting obscured. The best way for seniors to overcome this mental haze is to concentrate on topics that interest them or work on puzzles.

Cannabis may impair thinking to be less alert and coherent.

While THC can affect short-term memory, it does not affect recalling long-term memories. Seniors are not likely to forget their name or where they live while under the influence of cannabis, but they might get fuzzy on lesser significant details or while trying to recite states and capitals.

Scientists believe that when people ingest cannabis, their cannabinoid receptors work on regulating memory formation. They speculate that the receptors act as filters to prevent the mind from being flooded with information overload. Again, lowering dosage is the main way help seniors their comfort level.

Certain cannabis strains can make consumers more imaginative, which the reason many artists credit cannabis for their creativity. Other strains can make the mind rather cloudy, much like being in a dream state. Getting high on cannabis has various effects but the stereotype of pot smokers being foggy minded is true only for a minority, contrary to exaggerated arguments that helped shape 20th Century anti-pot propaganda.

Because cannabis is an intoxicant, it can impair thinking. It's possible, for example, for someone who has smoked a lot of cannabis to be less alert and coherent, which is why seniors under the influence of cannabis should avoid operating equipment or driving a vehicle.

Fortunately, memory can be improved in many ways whether cannabis is involved or not. Engaging in trivia games with friends is a fun, competitive way to strengthen memory. Reciting information internally several times also helps as does a notepad for jotting down thoughts and ideas. The important thing to remember is that cannabis only causes short term memory loss during the high and that CBD counters the memory loss effects of THC.

Increased Heart Rate

The relationship between cannabis and heart rate is not completely understood due to conflicting animal studies, but THC appears to be the cause of increased heart rate while CBD counters the effect. According to a study conducted by Donald P. Tashkin, M.D. at UCLA School of Medicine, long-term heavy cannabis use does not have an affect on contraction of the heart muscle, although it can cause a short-term increase in heart rate. *The Journal of the American Heart Association* warned that cannabis can trigger heart problems. It's important for seniors who may have cardiovascular issues to discuss their using cannabis with their personal physicians.

Medical experts agree that people who have suffered heart problems should be cautious about cannabis because it may speed heart rate.

Since heart conditions are a serious concern, it's imperative for seniors to consult their doctors before beginning cannabis therapy.

More research needs to be done to learn the relationship between cannabis and the cardiovascular system. Research is contradictory because cannabinoids have been shown to lower blood pressure and protect against nerve cell damage following a stroke.

Since heart conditions are a serious concern, it's imperative for seniors to consult their doctors before beginning cannabis therapeutics. For those who do use cannabis with cardiovascular issues, meditation is one of the keys to reducing heart rate along with using slow breathing exercises. Relaxation and positive thoughts help reduce anxiety or panic.

Cannabis is gaining the acceptance among medical professionals as a legitimate treatment. But it also has a few side effects that may concern seniors. The key is to be informed about cannabis and to learn from professionals who can help inform about the best strains and appropriate dosages with limited side effects. Much of the discomfort may be psychological, so keep in mind that self-confidence is a major factor in how seniors respond to cannabis.

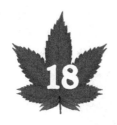

Cannabis Promotes Socializing

Seniors experience loneliness more than those in other ages groups. Seniors tend to spend large amounts of time alone. Some are widowed. Others have lost friends to death. Many seniors have reduced mobility, making it difficult to go places. Add in that many seniors live alone and it is easy to see why loneliness is an issue.

What is Loneliness?

Loneliness can be described as negative feelings or sadness brought on by a lack of communication, companionship or relationships with other people. Seniors are particularly vulnerable to feeling lonely. Eighteen percent of seniors live alone, while 43 percent report feeling lonely on a regular basis, according to a study conducted by researchers from the University of California, San Francisco. Lonely seniors are more likely to decline and die sooner. The UCSF study also found that people 60-years-old and older who reported

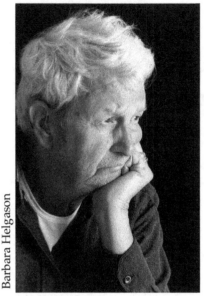

Barbara Helgason

Many seniors struggle with loneliness.

feeling lonely saw a 45 percent increase in their risk for death. Isolated elders also had a 59 percent greater risk of mental and physical decline than their more social counterparts.

Roots of Loneliness

Social contacts tend to decrease as we age for a variety of reasons, including retirement, the death of friends and family, or lack of mobility. Dr. Marc Agronin, medical director for mental health and clinical research at the Miami Jewish Health Systems, noted that one of the major causes of isolation is widowhood, particularly for couples who have had interdependent relationships. The same can be true for spouses whose partners have dementia or are chronically ill. Social contact can fade away if they're consumed with caregiving or no longer go out much.

Loneliness is Risky

Regardless of the causes of senior isolation, the consequences can be alarming and even harmful.

Feelings of loneliness can negatively affect both physical and mental health. Social isolation in seniors is linked to long-term illness and contributes to cognitive decline and risk of dementia. Loneliness in seniors is a major risk factor for depression. Studies have found that socially isolated seniors are twice as likely to die prematurely.

As people grow older they are more likely to lose loved ones, and may live alone. They are also more likely to experience health problems, which can make it harder to get out and about. All of these can increase feelings of loneliness and isolation. Many people experience loneliness either as a result of living alone, a lack of close family ties, reduced connections with their culture of origin or an inability to actively participate in the local community activities. When this occurs in combination with physical disablement, demoralization and depression are common accompaniments.

Loneliness is Self-Propelling

Loneliness is self-propelling. Older adults who feel lonely are more prone to behave in ways that may cause other people to not want to be around them. Psychologists from the University of Chicago who

Loneliness can be described as negative feelings or sadness brought on by a lack of communication, companionship or relationships with other people.

analyzed data from the Farmingham Heart Study, a long-term, ongoing cardiovascular study, found that solitary seniors have a tendency to further isolate themselves by pushing people away and not making efforts to engage with others.

Depressed seniors may find it challenging to get along with others, to "go with the flow" in social situations, and to maintain relationships. Many depressed seniors are incapable of being "good company" for friends and family. Some grow completely dissatisfied with relationships and withdraw from social interactions.

Cannabis Boosts Sociability

Cannabis is effective in soothing depression. Using cannabis can transform one's mental state. Often all that is needed is eating a cannabis edible, taking a "hit" from a pipe or a few drops of tincture under the tongue to improve mood and demeanor. A major plus of enjoying cannabis is that it has few, if any, side effects—a stark contrast to anti-depressant medications that often wreak havoc on the body and mind with nasty side effects.

Using cannabis breaks down the barriers to socialization. Introverted and depressed individuals who shy away from social interactions tend to feel more inclined to engage with others after using cannabis.

Silencing the Internal Critic

We often tend to be highly critical of ourselves. We are taught to think before speaking and to avoid saying anything controversial. Resulting from suspicion, shyness or depression, many seniors hesitate to interact with strangers because they have been conditioned to scrutinize thoughts, feelings and even verbalized statements after uttering them. Many do not even reach the point of verbalizing such thoughts because of being caught up in questioning their merit.

Using cannabis aids in silencing this internal critic. Social interacting is easier when not plagued by an internal critic's filter so that cannabis users are more inclined to interact with others and share their opinions. Conversation flows more freely, friendships are made and individuals enjoy uplifting social experiences. This is part of the magic of cannabis. Some seniors feel empowered to the point that they speak or act in a manner that reflects their uniqueness.

Divergent Thinking; Sharpened Senses

Studies on the effects of cannabis use have revealed a recurrent theme amongst cannabis users: divergent thinking—thinking quite irreverent yet extremely healthy. Divergent thinking is centered on making connections between seemingly unrelated concepts or thoughts. Using cannabis heightens such irreverent thought patterns, empowering individuals to partake in interesting conversations that often lead to lasting relationships.

Seniors who consume cannabis often find their senses heightened, with time passing slowly, audio stimulation sounding richer and colors appearing more vibrant. This heightened state of awareness makes just about everything more enjoyable. Depressed individuals who derive more enjoyment out of social interactions and group activities stand a greater chance of emerging from their negative mind state.

How to Facilitate Socializing

Seniors can get together to talk over a pipe, vaporizer or cannabis edibles. These "smoke circles" provide opportunities for social interaction while passing the cannabis from one person to the next.

Cannabis enthusiasts may get together to watch movies, play video games or board games, catch a sporting event or listen to music. Some enjoy cannabis in the midst of these get-togethers while others treat themselves to cannabis beforehand as a means of lubricating their social graces.

Group events known as "edible parties" are popular. Seniors come together to eat dose-specific edibles at such parties. Potluck style parties are popular where each reveler brings a cannabis edible to share with the rest of the group. Once the party-goers have consumed cannabis edibles, they partake in social activities with less reservation.

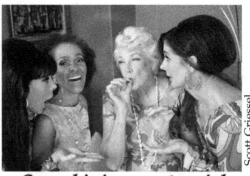

Scott Griessel

Cannabis is a great social facilitator for seniors.

Seniors suffering from loneliness find cannabis therapy to be helpful in being more outgoing and friendly. Using cannabis therapeutically is a kind of social lubricant that greases the wheels of interactions. Those who have tried cannabis testify that it improved their social experiences by putting them at ease and inspiring them to strike up conversations. Cannabis therapeutics may be a bridge that connects shy, inward seniors to new friends, which may last for years.

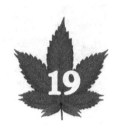

Healing Laughter

There is a proven benefit of cannabis that often goes overlooked—laughing. It is well-known that using cannabis can incite laughter, from quiet giggling to uncontrollable boisterous guffaws. But few realize such mirth actually has healing power. Laughing can improve mental well-being as well as having a beneficial impact on physical health. Laughter really is the best medicine.

Benefits of Laughing

When laughing, tension is released—much like an orgasm or sneezing does. Comedians use this well-known secret when they build up tension and then release it with a punch line.

Scientists say that a belly laugh has an opposite physiological response to that produced by stress, supporting that laughing is an eustress state producing positive emo-

> *Laughing is an eustress state producing positive emotions.*

tions. Research results indicate that, after laughing, there is an increase in activity within the immune system,

Many experts believe laughter is a behavior meant to help strengthen human connections.

including an increase in the activity level of killer cells and antibody action.

What Is Laughter?

There are a few different theories behind why we laugh. One is that laughter is an instinctual behavior incited by the shared relief of passing danger. The flight or flight response, which is a biological response shared by everyone, can be inhibited by a bout of laughter due to the fact that laughter relaxes a person. This, in turn, may show that laughter indicates trust in the people around you.

Many experts believe laughter is a behavior meant to help strengthen human connections, which strengthens the argument of it being a way to communicate. For example, the more you laugh with a group of people, the stronger your bond with those people grows. Not to mention that when a group of people laugh, it often causes you to laugh because laughing is "contagious".

What Happens When Laughing

Different parts of the brain are responsible for different functions, but laughter is unique in that

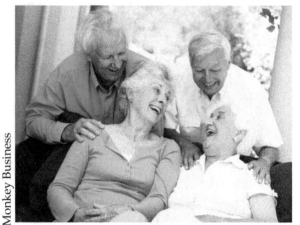

Monkey Business

After laughing for only a few minutes, you may feel better for hours.

laughter involves numerous parts of the brain. For example, emotional responses are a function of the frontal lobe, which is the biggest region of the brain. However, the left hemisphere of the cortex analyzes the situation that invokes the laughter, while the right hemisphere analyzes the situation in order to understand it. Additionally, the sensory processing area of the occipital lobe helps process visual signs, while the motor section of the brain is stimulated to evoke a physical response.

Laughter helps you feel better about yourself and the world around you. Laughter is a natural diversion. When laughing, other thoughts are briefly blocked. Laughing can also induce physical changes in the body. After laughing for only a few minutes, you may feel better for hours. The biggest benefit of laughter is that it is free and has no known negative side effects.

Laughing Back to Health

It was 1964 when journalist Norman Cousins was diagnosed with *Ankylosing Spondylitis*, a rare disease of the connective tissues and told he had a 1 in 500 chance of surviving more than a few months. Being a fighter, Cousins rejected the diagnosis and instead used his journalism skills to research medical journals. He discovered that his disease and the medicines he was taking were both depleting his body of vitamin C.

He found a new doctor and began to get injections of massive doses of vitamin C. Then he got a movie projector and a box of funny movies, like the Marx Brothers, which he watched for hours. In spite of the constant pain, Cousin pushed himself to laugh until his very stomach hurt from it. Miraculously Cousins lived through November 1990, surviving 26 years longer than doctors had predicted.

Laughter has therapeutic value in fighting disease, including cancer.

While it can't be proven that laughing added years to Norman Cousins' life, a growing body of research supports the theory that laughter has therapeutic value in fighting disease, including cancer.

7 Humor Habits

Studies show that practicing the 7 Humor Habits boosts positive emotions and subjective well-being.

- Surround yourself with humor
- Cultivate a playful attitude
- Laugh more often and more heartily
- Create your own verbal humor
- Look for humor in every day life
- Take yourself lightly; laugh at yourself
- Find humor in the midst of stress

McGhee, Paul. *Humor: The Lighter Path to Resilience and Health.* Author House, 2010

A study showed that stress constricts blood vessels and suppresses immune activity and that these responses decreased in subjects who were exposed to humor. Levels of epinephrine were lower in the group both in anticipation of humor and after exposure to humor. Laughing is aerobic, providing a workout for the diaphragm, increasing the body's ability to use oxygen.

Laughter Therapy

Experts believe that when used as an adjunct to conventional medical care, laughter can reduce pain and aid the healing process. In a study published in the *Journal of Holistic Nursing*, patients listened to one-liners after surgery and before painful medication was administered. Subjects exposed to humor reported experiencing less pain when compared to patients who didn't get a dose of humor as part of their therapy.

Now days many hospitals such as Cancer Treatment Centers of America (CTCA) include laughter therapy in their treatment protocol. CTCA offers humor therapy sessions—known as "Laughter Clubs"—to help cancer patients and their families use laughter as a tool for healing. These leader-led groups take patients through a number of laugh-related exercises including fake laughter and laughter greetings. It is hard for people not to join in because laughter is so contagious. Dr. Katherine Puckett, National Director of Mind-Body Medicine at the CTCA in Chicago, says cancer patients find that laughing out loud, especially in a group setting, can help them through their cancer journey.

Laughter appears to change brain chemistry as well as boosting the immune system. Some speculate that humor allows a person to feel in control of a disease, making it seem more manageable. For one thing, laughter offers a powerful distraction from pain. Laughing enables the release

Experts believe that when used as an adjunct to conventional medical care, laughter can reduce pain and aid the healing process.

fears, anger, and stress—all of which can harm the body over time. Humor improves the quality of life.

Laughter offers a physical benefit. Researchers estimate that laughing a hundred times has roughly the equal physical value as 15 minutes on an exercise bike. Laughing works out parts of the body, such as the diaphragm, the abdominal muscles, the respiratory muscles, the facial muscles, the back muscles and even the leg muscles.

Cannabis Encourages Mirth

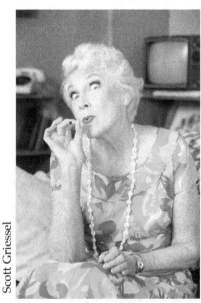

Scott Griessel

Laughing 100 times is roughly equal to 15 minutes on an exercise bike.

Studies have shown that using cannabis stimulates flow of blood to the right frontal and left temporal lobes, two areas that are associated with laughter—making it easier to produce laughter. Additionally cannabis has been linked to the promotion of neurogenesis in the brain to help fight anxiety and depression, making it easier to experience positive emotions.

Using cannabis is often social—passing around a joint or bong, encourages laughing. Some strains of cannabis are more effective at promoting laughter. Strains, like linalool and limonene, contain terpenes that work to elevate moods, offer stress relief, soothe anxiety, and fight depression.

Smoking tends to cause more of a head high and is considered the most social way to consume cannabis, since a joint or vape can be passed around in a group encouraging conviviality. The more cannabis consumption is a social experience, the more potential for laughter to ignite due to its contagious nature.

Consuming cannabis through edibles is the second most popular method of use. Even though it takes about an hour for effects to "come on", they generally last longer than when smoking, which means you could extend longer periods of laughter.

Cannabis doesn't automatically promote laughter as soon as it's consumed. The proper dosage is needed to ensure healthy laughter. A dose that's too small may not result in a mental state that's strong enough, while a

Smoking tends to cause more of a head high and is considered the most social way to consume cannabis, since a joint or vape can be passed around in a group encouraging conviviality.

dose that's too large may trigger anxiety instead of mirth.

With edibles, it is generally best to keep the dosage at a moderate level to encourage robust laughter. If the dose is too small—you can nibble a bit more of the cookie or brownie—but not too much. Remember: less is best. Avoid giving in to the "munchies"—a common side effect of using cannabis—because eating can cause the effects of cannabis to wear off sooner.

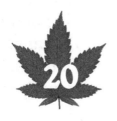

20

Cannabis Topicals

Topical cannabis is gaining popularity, especially for those who do not want to inhale or swallow cannabis. Topicals such as lotions, patches, or ointments are applied directly on the skin where they offer location-specific relief. The cannabinoids within are absorbed through the skin into the body, avoiding the bloodstream. Dosages can be controlled easily in order to avoid over- or under-doing it.

Topical cannabis is often preferred by seniors

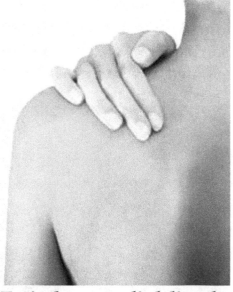

Topicals are applied directly on the skin where they offer location-specific relief.

because they are easy to administer and offer a more controlled method of delivery. Many cannabis topicals contain 100 cannabidiol (CBD), a non-psychoactive cannabinoid. By administering a CBD lotion or transdermal patch, there is no risk of getting the "high" associated with THC, which may still be in CBD-dominant strains. Topicals are simple to make at home, allowing each individual to create a natural salve or lotion that is specifically designed for their unique needs.

How Topicals Work

Topical cannabis treatments penetrate the CB2 receptors within the endocannabinoid system. However, without a carrier agent such as oleic acid, they will not penetrate the blood/brain barrier, which is how the "high" of THC is avoided. Cannabinoids have easy access to the

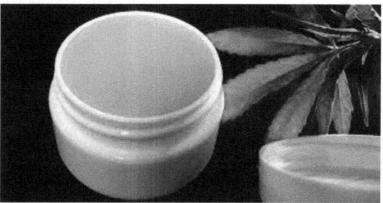

Topical cannabis treatments penetrate the CB2 receptors within the endocannabinoid system.

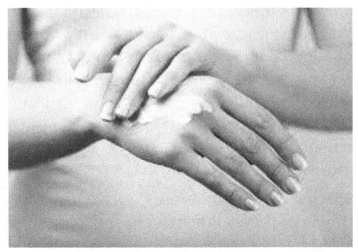

Topical cannabis treatments are applied directly to the problem area, offering fast-acting and efficient relief.

CB2 receptors through pores and hair follicles, making them efficient when it comes to treating location-specific issues like muscle pain and skin disorders. There is no need to metabolize or break through the blood/brain barrier. The cannabinoids stay right where they are applied.

When smoking cannabis, the cannabinoids travel through the lungs to get the bloodstream. Edibles pass through the intestines before the cannabinoids are sent to blood. The issue with these delivery methods is that cannabinoids travel through the body before they reach the intended target. Topical cannabis treatments are applied directly to the problem area, offering fast-acting and efficient relief.

Cannabis lotions, salves, transdermal patches and other topicals can be used to treat a variety of ailments. Burns, skin imperfections, stiff muscles/joints, localized pain, and bacterial/fungal infections are some of the most common issues treated with topicals. There is growing popularity in using topical cannabis to treat arthritis and psoriasis.

Specific cannabinoids are typically used for the treatment of these ailments. The most common is CBD, which has shown efficacy as an anti-inflammatory, analgesic, and treatment for psoriasis. Both THC and CBD are used as anti-fungals. The lesser known cannabinoids CBC and CBG are known for their ability to slow bacteria growth, making them the perfect choice for treating skin infections. It is important to note that the majority of cannabinoids do not get the user "high," with the exception of THC.

Transdermal Topicals

Transdermal patches containing cannabinoids work differently from lotions, salves, or ointments because they contain carrier agents, which allow penetration through blood/brain barrier. Transdermal delivery offers an advantageous mode of cannabinoid administration by eliminating first pass metabolism and providing sustained release for a prolonged period of time that can be controlled by the individual. Transdermal cannabis creates more of a body high but is not like that of an edible high—edibles last much longer and can be more intense whereas transdermal cannabis penetrates slowly to offer subtle, long-lasting symptom relief.

Transdermal cannabis patches are often used to treat muscle pain/aches, nausea and inflammation. By penetrating all layers of the skin, patches can reach the affected area quickly and directly. They can be left on for several hours, offering relief in a discreet manner all day long. Seniors who play sports or engage in other physical activities may choose to use transdermal cannabis patches for maintenance during their exercise much like those who opt for traditional pain patches.

Versatile and Targeted

Topical cannabis treatments are an excellent way to treat specific areas of the body in a way that prevents the typical "high" of smoking, vaporizer, or eating marijuana. Lotions, salves, ointments, and transdermal patches deliver cannabinoids to the CB2 receptor for location-specific relief.

Topicals can be used to treat everything from muscle aches and pains to psoriasis of the skin. Making cannabis-infused topicals at home is simple and gives people the opportunity to have complete control over ingredients and dosages.

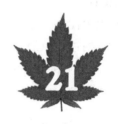

Cooking with Cannabis

Seniors who desire the benefits of cannabis therapeutics but do not want to smoke or vaporize cannabis can turn to cannabis edibles. Cannabis is primarily infused into food through butter and oils. When you've mastered the art of making a great bud-butter or bud-oil, you can cook cannabis into virtually anything calling for these ingredients.

The canna-butter or canna-oil is simply substituted in dishes that would call for regular oil or butter. Delicious! You can add cannabis to any food that contains animal or vegetable fats, such as cakes, biscuits, stews or drinks such as milk shakes, drinking chocolate or yoghurt.

> *The canna-butter or canna-oil is simply substituted in dishes that would call for regular oil or butter. Delicious!*

Though it takes longer for the therapeutic effects of cannabis to manifest when consumed in an edible as opposed to smoking or vaporizing, it is well worth the wait. Cannabis edibles do everything from relieving pain to calming the nerves and inducing a restful sleep.

Benefits for Seniors

A growing number of senior citizens are relying on cannabis edibles for pain management, anxiety relief and even as a sleep aid. Most seniors do not want to use a pipe or vaporizer to inhale burned or baked cannabis. Nor do they want to add another pain or sleeping pill to their daily pill intake. It is much easier to chow down on a delicious cannabis edible.

Unlike sleeping pills and many pain medications, cannabis edibles are not addictive. Add in the fact that cannabis edibles have few side effects

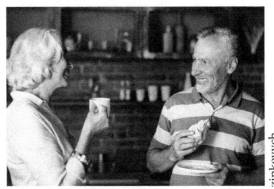

Cannabis edibles are not addictive.

zinkevych

compared to pain medications and it is easy to understand why so many seniors are turning to these tasty treats. A rough rule of thumb is to select indica dominant strains for cramping and muscle spasticity and sativa dominant strains for mental pick up.

There is a danger lurking in these yummy edibles and it is the sugar. Cannabis edibles are especially helpful with pain and arthritis management. Countless seniors graze on cannabis edibles throughout the day to reduce chronic pain that would otherwise limit their functionality.

Plenty of seniors also find cannabis edibles helpful in their quest for a solid night's sleep. Many seniors find it difficult to achieve restful sleep as they are plagued by pain. Some seniors suffer from limited mobility that prevents them from being active during the day. Idle seniors often find it difficult to sleep for eight hours each night, yet those who turn to cannabis edibles in the hours before bedtime stand a greater chance of reaching the coveted REM sleep stage that allows them to wake up feeling refreshed.

It is also worth noting that cannabis edibles are quite economical as compared to traditional pain medications. There is no sense in paying thousands of dollars per year for an array of pain pills when one can spend hundreds or less on cannabis edibles. This savings is especially important for seniors on fixed incomes.

A note of caution: There is a tendency to make sugary edibles, like cookies, cakes, brownies. There is a danger lurking in these yummy edibles and it is the sugar. High sugar diets promote many terrible disorders, like cancer, diabetes, obesity, and heart disease. It is hard to do, but keep sugary edibles to a minimum and concentrate on using the canna-oil in salads, fried eggs, soups, and bread.

Infusing Cannabinoids

Some marijuana food recipes use finely ground cannabis but this makes for a rather crunchy experience that some likened to a cow chewing its cud. More importantly, however, is that it is inefficient because the cannabinoids remain bound up in the plant during the digestion process and are excreted along with the roughage, so most of the pot is wasted. THC is easily released by smoking but THC is not readily digested. It must be extracted into a form that the body can metabolize. The best approach is to extract the cannabinoids from the plant. Because cannabinoids are solvable in oil and alcohol, but not water, oil and alcohol are used to extract the essence from the cannabis.

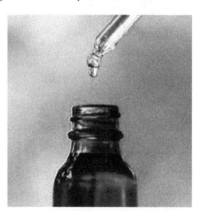

Infuse cannabis into alcohol for a tincture.

Cannabinoids can infuse into alcohol for a tincture that is placed on or beneath the tongue with an eyedropper. Others elect to make home-made vaporizer oils for oral ingestion. Infusing cannabis into butter that is used in edibles is the most popular way to consume cannabis in food form. This cannabis butter is commonly referred to as "canna-butter" or "ghee". It is best to use an oil with a particularly high fat content. Oils that are not derived from genetically modified crops are desirable. Furthermore, the best cannabis-infused oils aren't excessively refined. If the oil is highly refined, it will make the cannabis extraction process that much more challenging.

Lipids

While cannabis lipids can be added to just about any food item, they are ideal for foods that are baked. When cannabis is extracted, it gravitates towards lipids that are then used in the cooking process. The key is to find recipes that make use of fats and oils like butter. Canna-oils and canna-butter are then substituted for those traditional oils/fats. THC extraction occurs with fats like butter, bacon fat, olive oil, coconut oil and avocado oil.

Lipids are ideal for baked foods.

As long as the fat is heated together with the cannabis, cannabinoids will disperse into the lipids. This relationship is replicated in the person's body when the cannabis-infused food is consumed.

Butter, being a saturated fat, can pose health issues.

Though there is some disagreement over which particular fats are the best for extracting THC from cannabis, anecdotal claims point to butter, coconut oil and bacon fat as ideal. Butter is by far the most popular fat for cannabis cooking. However, butter does not retain cannabinoids as easily as certain oils such as coconut oil.

Dairy products like heavy cream absorb and hold cannabinoids with ease yet they are also prone to burning. Those who decide to use dairy products for cannabis extraction will need considerable patience. This extraction process takes hours and the constant attention of the cook. When in doubt, use coconut oil. It is the premier oil for cannabinoid infusion as it is versatile and retains more cannabinoids than most other oils/fats. Once the cannabis is extracted, the resulting oil can either be ingested or applied in a topical manner.

Another issue with butter, being a saturated fat, is that it can pose health issues. Olive oil is considered to be among the healthiest oils due to its high content of monounsaturated fatty acids and its high content of antioxidative substances. Olive oil has anti-inflammatory properties. Most people do quite well with it since it does not upset the critical omega 6 to omega 3 ratio and most of the fatty acids in olive oil are actually an omega-9 oil, which is monounsaturated. Some people don't like the taste of olive oil. You can experiment with other anti-inflammatory oils, which include coconut oil and almond oil.

Decarboxilation

Decarboxilation is a cannabis toasting or baking process that brings about the plant's inherent neuroprotective and anti-inflammatory qualities. This process makes it possible for cannabis to work its magic. If cannabis were consumed without decarboxilation, it would not make much of an impact on the human body and mind. Decarboxilation requires that the cannabis be dried, cured and toasted or baked. Those who smoke or vaporize their cannabis perform the decarboxilation process when they burn/bake the plant with their lighters/vaporizer baking spaces. A similar

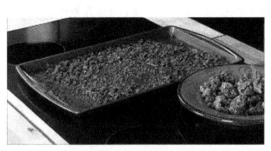

process must happen to cannabis before it can work its magic in edible form.

A temperature of at least 220 degrees is required for cannabis decarboxilation.

Cannabis should be heated at a fairly

low temperature over time so it can be infused in an effective manner. A temperature of at least 220 degrees is required for cannabis decarboxilation.

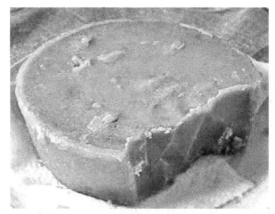

Bud-butter can be substituted for butter or oil in almost any recipe.

It should be baked at this temperature for about half an hour. A comprehensive decarboxilation might require upwards of 45 minutes of baking time. A temperature in excess of 300 degrees Fahrenheit will harm the integrity of cannabinoids as well as terpenoids.

Bud-Butter

Bud-butter, which is THC extracted into butter, is the basic cannabis cooking ingredient. Bud-butter can be substituted for the call for butter or oil in almost any recipe. If you fry breakfast eggs in butter, try using a teaspoon of bud-butter as your frying medium. People on anti-inflammatory diets to reduce pain, should use canola oil for extraction, because butter is an inflammatory food that can trigger migraines and arthritis flair ups in sensitive people.

Potency

When using the best Grade A cannabis indica, use a ratio of 1 ounce of cannabis to 16-20 ounces of bud-butter. This will yield 100-125 teaspoons of very potent extract. When using Grade B cannabis, use a ratio of one ounce of cannabis to 8 ounces of butter to yield 50 teaspoons of extract. With Grade C cannabis you'll need to use a high cannabis-to-butter ratio, such as one ounce of cannabis to 4 ounces of butter. With canna-butter made from seeds and stems, use an especially high ratio of cannabis to butter.

Storing Bud-Butter

It is best to make only as much bud-butter as you need for a particular recipe because it can get stale and go rancid. However, it is convenient to have prepared bud-butter on hand, especially if you are cooking for only one or two. One great method is to freeze it in ice cube trays. Each cube will be approximately ¼ cup of bud-butter. When a recipe calls for ½ cup of butter, you simply pop out two cubes and drop into your recipe.

> *It is best to make only as much bud-butter as you need for a particular recipe because it can get stale and go rancid.*

How to Make Bud Cooking Oil

Ingredients:

- 48 oz bottle canola cooking oil
- Large-sized cooking pot
- 1 oz of cannabis buds
- Metal strainer

Pour canola oil into the cooking pot. Heat on medium until hot. Do not allow to boil. Crumble cannabis indica into small bits and add to hot oil. Stir oil herb mixture every ten minutes for two hours. If the mixture starts to boil remove from heat and let cool and turn burner heat down.

Mind the Dosage

When cooking with cannabis, it is not prudent to replace a recipe's suggested amount of oil or butter with cannabis-infused oil or butter. Start out with a fairly small amount of cannabis-infused butter or oil. Use a third or half of the recipe's suggested amount and round out the remainder with traditional oil or butter. See what type of effects this dose brings about and adjust accordingly with future recipes. In terms of recipes, some of the most popular cannabis-infused foods are brownies, cookies, rice krispie treats, macaroni and cheese, biscuits, caramels and salad dressings. Again, be watchful of the amount of sugar you consume.

Masking the Cannabis Flavor

Though many seniors desire the positive effects of cannabis-infused foods, a good portion of them dislike the taste and smell of cannabis. The solution is to use cannabis-infused oils and butters with foods that mask the flavor of cannabis. Examples of such foods or herbs include mint, chocolate, peanut butter, rosemary, garlic, parsley, basil and fruit flavors like mango and papaya.

Complementing Cannabis Flavor

Certain foods make the cannabis flavor more palatable. Though taste buds differ by individual, plenty of seniors are partial to specific dishes and flavors with their cannabis. Examples include salmon with lemony cannabis strains and lemon bars with fruity strains to balance the citrus. Others are partial to lemon-pepper chicken, teriyaki chicken, Hawaiian pizza, steak, fish with vegetables, spinach and strawberry salad, ice cream and chocolate chip cookies.

Cannabis cooking is poised to take center stage as it becomes socially normative in the years to come. It won't be long until cannabis cooking shows are featured on TV and the web. Cannabis restaurants are popping up in select cities throughout the nation. Anyone who is on the prowl for a way to enjoy the many therapeutic effects of cannabis without smoking or vaporizing the plant should give cannabis cooking a try.

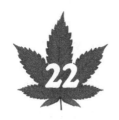
22

DIY Cannabis Medicines

It is relatively easy for seniors to make their own cannabis medicines right in their kitchens at home.

Compresses and Poultices

A compress is a pad of absorbent material infused with medicine, then pressed onto the painful part of the body to relieve inflammation. A compress can be any temperature—cold, lukewarm, or hot. It can be wet or dry. When you have pain related to muscle fatigue, a painful carbuncle, or a shiver in your bones, a warm compress can make you feel much better.

Wet Compress

Saturate a washcloth with cannabis oil. Fold the wet cloth and place it in a plastic bag with

A compress is a pad of absorbent material infused with medicine, then pressed onto the painful part of the body to relieve inflammation.

a zip closure, leaving the bag open. Put in a microwave oven and heat on High for 30-60 seconds. Remove the hot washcloth and bag from microwave carefully, and place it on a dry towel. Close the bag. Wrap the towel around the baggie in such a way that it won't slide out and there is a layer of towel between the hot washcloth and your skin.

Place the warm compress over the aching area and leave for about 10 minutes. Remove and allow the area to cool. Reheat the washcloth and repeat.

Poultices

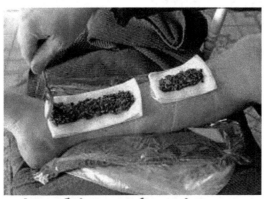

A poultice a soft, moist mass of material, typically of plant material or flour, applied to the body to relieve soreness and inflammation and kept in place with a cloth.

A poultice is a soft, mushy preparation composed of a pulpy or mealy herbal substance that can absorb a large amount of fluid. The herbal matter is mashed into a paste using hot liquids and spread thickly on a cloth and applied, while hot, to the painful or inflamed area if the body. Poultices work through moist heat, which must be renewed after several minutes or otherwise kept warm. The cloth can then be covered with plastic wrap to hold in the moisture.The poultice should be changed whenever it dries out.

A poultice can be used to draw out infection, treat boils and abscesses, relieve inflammation or a rash or simply draw the poison from a bee sting!

Seniors can soak cannabis leaves in alcohol and apply them as a poultice to an arthritic or swollen joint. Poultices can be used to heal bruises, break up congestion, reduce inflammation, withdraw pus from putrid sores, soothe abrasions, or withdraw toxins from an area. They may be applied hot or cold, depending on the health need. Cold poultices are used to withdraw the heat from an inflamed or congested area. Use a hot poultice to relax spasms and for some pains.

A compress is used the same way but usually warm liquids are applied to the cloth instead of raw substances. Tinctures or herbal infusions are great for compresses.

How to Make a Poultice

If you are using fresh cannabis, mix half a cup of the herbs with one cup of water in a saucepan and simmer it for two minutes. With dried can nabis, simply mix it with warm water to make a paste. Pour the mixture onto a piece of cloth and apply it to the affected area. Then secure the gauze or cloth with a bandage or towel.

Cannabis Poultice

Ingredients

- 2-3 tablespoons (or more as needed) of fresh or dried cannabis, healing clays or activated charcoal as needed
- Enough hot water to form a thick paste
- Organic cheesecloth or cloth for covering
- Waterproof covering upon which to put the poultice.

Instructions

Make a thick paste with the desired herb, clay or charcoal and water. Apply directly to the wound or place between two layers of cloth and apply the cloth to the wound—depending on the cloth and the wound. Leave for 20 minutes to 3 hours as needed and repeat as necessary.

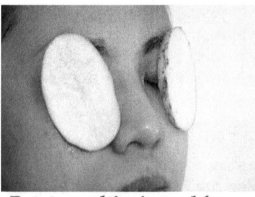

Potato poultice is good for eye inflammation.

Potato Poultice

Grate a raw potato and make your paste! A potato poultice is good for inflammation and eye troubles such as conjunctivitis.

Mustard Poultice

Mash some mustard seeds, mix with natural oil or water and apply. Use thin cloth between paste and skin. A homemade mustard poultice is very powerful and can burn your skin if applied directly.

Topical Cannabis Liniment

Ingredients

- 3-7 g. cannabis leaf, ground fine
- Rubbing alcohol

Grind cannabis into a fine powder. Pour about 1/3 bottle of rubbing alcohol into a separate container for future use. Using a funnel, pour the ground cannabis into the bottle. Shake well, then store in a dark place. Shake daily, for 1-2 months. Using a cloth strain out solid material. Apply liberally to affected area for pain relief, as needed. Good for arthritis, and muscle pain.

Salves and Balms

Salve is a broad term used to describe lotions, ointments, pastes, and creams that soothe or heal an area of the body that is excessively dry, irritated, burned, or wounded. In many cases, salves contain natural ingredients that can promote the healing process and reduce discomfort in the area being treated.

> *In many cases, salves contain natural ingredients that can promote the healing process and reduce discomfort in the area being treated.*

They are commonly used to treat severely dry hands, chapped lips, and sunburned skin. cannabis salves have been used to relieve muscle aches and pains for generations. They relieve topical pain and can be used in combination with other herbs. However, salves can be messy.

Prepare a salve by using coconut oil and cannabis and cooking in the same fashion as when making bud-butter. Adding other medicinal plants like aloe, comfrey, yarrow, ginger can greatly help with the healing qualities. The more plant material the better. Cool overnight. Then separate the oil from the water. Heat the oil again to boil off any additional water and pour into a glass jar.

Apply the salve to area with pain, spasm, or damage. Use a nice amount but don't try to over-saturate area. For best results, apply after a hot shower.

Medicated Cannabis Salve

Ingredients:

- 4 cups olive oil
- 1 cup St. Johns wort
- 2 cups dried calendula blossoms
- 1/4 cup comfrey root
- 1/4 cup lavender flowers
- 6 tbsp coconut oil
- 1 1/2 cups dried cannabis leaf
- 2 -3 tbsp beeswax

Heat the oils and add the dried roots and keep just below the simmer point. If you see bubbles then turn down the heat. Steep the herbs for 2 to 3 hours, stirring every once in awhile. Cool and strain using a cloth. Place in a clean bowl and add beeswax.

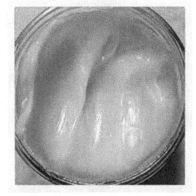

Other oils, like hemp oil, can be substituted or added along with various medicinal dried herbs and plant oils. The salve is great for bug bites, stings and scratches.

Salves are lotions, ointments, pastes, and creams that soothe or heal an area of the body

Quick Headache Salve

Ingredients

- Cannabis leaf infused olive oil
- Vitamin E (to help with absorption)
- Organic beeswax

Instructions

Use a double boiler to keep a low heat, if not, you can use a spare 1L. glass jar in a pot of water.

- Melt 1 1/3 Cups of organic beeswax (shaved if possible)
- Warm 2 Cups of infused Massage Oil
- Add 25 ml. Vit E. Oil to the massage Oil
- Stir well
- Add Melted Beeswax
- Stir very Well
- Allow to cool slightly
- Carefully pour into jars
- Makes approx. 16 4 oz. Jars

Hemp Salve

One of the most powerful hemp preparations is the hemp salve. Its efficiency was proven in the 1950's at the Olomouc University Hospital, where Prof. Jan Kabelik carried out his famous research on the antibacterial effects of cannabis indica.

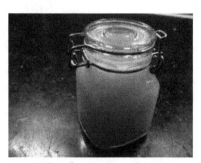

The hemp salve is a universal healing preparation.

One of the hospital pathologists cut his finger during an autopsy. Bacteria resistant to antibiotics infected the wound. Someone asked Prof. Kabelik for help because of his research on the medical use of cannabis. Hemp salve was applied to the infected wound and two days later the wound was healing. Amputation was avoided.

Vaseline is a good salve base for people suffering from allergies, although it does not penetrate as well as other bases.

The hemp salve is a universal healing preparation with multiple effects, combining the effects of an antibiotic ointment with the soothing effects of a salve to efficiently relieve arthritic and rheumatism pains. It is very efficient for the treatment of burns, certain eczemas, psoriasis and fungus. Never use the salve on bleeding wounds.

Hemp Salve

Ingredients:

- 1 jar Vaseline
- 100 g. cannabis leaves, crushed or
- 50 g. cannabis buds, crushed

Melt half of the Vaseline in a large pot, add cannabis and cook slowly for 20 minutes. Cool the mixture. Add 4 gallons water, bring to the boiling point, and slowly cook for 2 hours. Cool and refrigerate overnight. Take out the fatty cake and press to eliminate the water. Spread the cake on a cookie sheet, cover it and let it ferment for 3 weeks in a dark place at room temperature.

Put the mixture into a large pot and add the second half of Vaseline and melt it. Slowly cook the mixture until the fermentation smell dissipates. Strain through a strainer and pour the resulting green liquid into the top of a double boiler with water in the lower pan. Add finely crushed buds and cook in the water bath for an hour, stirring frequently. A light skim will form on the surface. Cool the mixture and store in a cool, dark place for a week to 10 days. Cook again in the top of a double boiler in water. Store the mixture in a dark, cool place for a week or so.

Again melt and cook the mixture as in the top of the double boiler. Strain through a strainer and then through a cloth. Pour the salve into small cosmetic jars.

Arthritis Balm

Ingredients

- 4 oz cannabis leaf
- Water
- 1 1/4 cup hemp oil
- 1-2 oz beeswax

Put cannabis in a large stock pot, cover with water and add hemp oil. Bring to a boil and simmer at a low boil for 5-6 hours, adding water as needed. Allow to cool and strain through cloth, saving the liquid. Place the liquid into the refrigerator over night. Peel the hemp oil layer off the top and place into a small pot and melt over low heat. Add beeswax, mix well, and cool into a salve.

Cannabis-Castor Oil Pack

Mix bud-oil and castor oil for a pack to fight inflammation, to help carpal tunnel syndrome or to soothe a strain. Apply the cannabis-caster oil to a cloth and place it on the injured area, like your wrist. Cover the area with plastic wrap. Place another rag on top of the plastic wrap and apply a heating pad for 30-45 minutes. The cannabis-castor oil is absorbed through the skin and help to reduce the inflammation in a very powerful way.

Essential Oils

Essential oils can also be added to homemade cannabis topicals, offering extra health benefits and a pleasant scent. There are many essential oils to choose from, all with unique properties that give different effects.

Lavender oil is known for its anti-inflammatory, relaxing effects while lemon oil is excellent as an antiseptic and energy booster. Musky oils such as patchouli and myrrh are often used as astringents. Is it important to remember not to apply essential oils directly on the skin—they must be diffused in topicals or water before touching the skin

Bibliography

Bar-Sela, G., Vorobeichik, M., Drawsheh, S., Omer, A., Goldberg, V., and Muller, E. (2013). *The Medical Necessity for Medicinal Cannabis: Prospective, Observational Study Evaluating the Treatment in Cancer Patients on Supportive or Palliative Care.* Evidence-Based Complementary and Alternative Medicine, 2013.

Bernhard, Toni. *How To Live Well With Chronic Pain and Illness: A MIndful Guide*, Wisdom Publicaitons, 2015.

Booth, M. *Cannabis: A History.* London, England: Picador, 2005.

Botek, Anne-Marie. *The Elder Loneliness Epidemic*, AgingCare.com.

Bradford, Ashley, & W. David Bradford. Marijuana Laws Reduce Prescription Medication Use In Medicare Part D. *Health Affairs*, vol. 35 no. 7, July, 2016, 1230-1236.

Brisbois, T.D., de Kock, I.H., Watanabe, S.M., Mirhosseini, M., Lamoureux, D.C., Chasen, M., MacDonald, N., Baracos, V.E., and Wismer, W.V. (2011, February 22). Delta-9-tetrahydrocannabinol may palliate altered chemosensory perception in cancer patients: results of a randomized-double-ble-blind, placebo-controlled pilot trial. *Annals of Oncolgy*, 22, 2086-2093.

Brownstein, Joe, Marijuana vs. Alcohol: Which Is Really Worse for Your Health? *LifeScience*, January, 2014.

Burstein, S.H., and Zurier, R.B. (2009, March). Cannabinoids, endocannabinoids, and related analogs in inflammation. *The AAPS Journal*, 11(1), 109-19.

Cannabis and Cannabinoids (PDQ). (2015, July 15). National Cancer Institute.

Challapalli PV, & AL. Stinchcomb. In vitro experiment optimization for measuring tetrahydrocannabinol skin permeation. *Int J Pharm*. 2002; 241:329–39.

Chemo side effects. (2015, June 9). American Cancer Society.

Chemotherapy Side Effects Worksheet. (n.d). American Cancer Society.

Choi, Charles Q., Why Marijuana Impairs Memory, *LifeScience*, Nov. 2006.

Corey-Bloom, J. & T. Wolfson, A. Gamst, S. Jin, TD Marcotte, H. Bentley, B. Gluaux. Smoked cannabis for spasticity in multiple sclerosis: a randomized, placebo-controlled trial. *CMAJ*, 2012 Jul 10;184(10):1143-50.

Costa, B., Colleoni, M., Conti, S., Parolaro, D., Franke, C., Trovato, A.E., and Giagnoni, G. (2004, March). Oral anti-inflammatory activity of cannabidiol, a non-psychoactive constituent of cannabis, in acute carrageenan-induced inflammation in the rat paw. *Naunyn-Schmiedeberg's Achives of Pharmacology*, 369(3), 294-9.

Cousins, Norman, *Head First: The Biology of Hope and the Healing Power of the Human Spirit*, Penguin Books, 1990.

Currais, Antonio. & Oswald Quehenberger, Aaron M. Armando, Daiel Daugherty, Pam Maher, & David Schubert. Amyloid proteotoxicity initiates an inflammatory response blocked by cannabinoids, *NPJ: Aging and Mechanisms of Disease*, June 2016.

Dahl, Melissa. Before Getting High, You Must First Learn How to Get High, *Science of US*, July, 2014.

Deitch, R. *Hemp: The Plant with a Divided History*. New York, NY: Algora Publishing, 2003.

Deardorff, William W. Opening and Closing the Pain Gates for Chronic Pain, *Spine-Health*, March 2003.

Esposito, Lisa. Silent Epidemic: Seniors and Addiction. *U.S.News*, December, 2015.

Gaffal E, & M. Cron, N. Glodde, T. Tuting. Anti-inflammatory activity of topical THC in DNFB-mediated mouse allergic contact dermatitis independent of CB1 and CB2 receptors. *Allergy,* 2013; 68: 994–1000.

Gouin, JP, & J. Kiecoult-Glaser. The Impact of Psychological Stress on Wound Healing: Methods and Mechanisms. *Immunology & Allergy Clinics of North America,* 2011, 31(1): 81-93.

Hampson, AJ. & M. Grimaldki, M. Lolic, D. Wink, R. Rosenthal, J. Axelrond. Neuroprotective Antioxidants from Marijuana. *Ann N Y Acad Sci.* 2000; 899: 274-82.

Health Editor, Almost All U.S. Doctors Are Overprescribing Narcotic Painkillers, Research Suggests, *Health Day News,* March, 2016.

Hutmacher, Abby. Why-Does-Marijuana-Make-Me-Dizzy? *Colorado Pot Guide.* Sep. 2015.

Hutmacher, A., & L. Thompson, & P. Staff. The Positive Effects of Cannabinoids. *Colorado Pot Guides,* 2016.

Jatoi, A., Windschitl, H.E., Loprinzi, C.L., Sloan, J.A., Dakhil, S.R., Mailliard, J.A., Pundaleeka, S., Kardinal, C.G., Fitch, T.R., Krook, J.E., Novotny, P.J. and Christensen, B. (2002). Dronabinol versus megestrol acetate versus combination therapy for cancer-associated anorexia: a North Central Cancer Treatment Group study. *Journal of Clinical Oncology,* 20(2), 567-73.

Jiang, Wen, Yun Zhang, Lan XIAO, Jamie Van Cleemput, Shao-Ping Ji, Guang Bai, and Xia Zhang. Cannabinoids promote embryonic and adult hippocampus neurogenesis and produce anxiolytic- and antidepressant-like effects, *Journal of Clinical Investigation,* Nov 2005.

Johnson, J.R., Burnell-Nugent, M., Lossignol, D., Ganae-Motan, E.D., Potts, R., and Fallon, M.T. (2010, February). Multicenter, double-blind, randomized, placebo-controlled, parallel-group study of the efficacy, safety, and tolerability of THC: CBD extract and THC extract in patients with intractable cancer-related pain. *Journal of Pain and Symptom Management,* 39(2), 167-79.

Jorge LL, & CC. Feres, VE. Teles. Topical preparations for pain relief: efficacy and patient adherence. *Journal of Pain Research*. 2011;4:11-24.

Kaye, A., & A. Baluch, J. Scott, J. Pain Management in the Elderly Population: A Review. *The Ochsner Journal*, 2010, 10(3): 179–187.

Klein, Allen, *The Healing Power of Humor: Techniques for Getting Through Loss, Setbacks, Upsets, Disappointments, Difficulties, Trials, Tribulations, and All That Not-So-Funny Stuff,* Tarcher/Putnam, 1989.

Joy, Janet E., Stanley J. Watson, Jr., and John A. Benson, Jr., Editors, *Marijuana and Medicine: Assessing the Science Base,* National Academy Press. 1999.

Lee, M. Amygdala activity contributes to the dissociative effect of cannabis on pain perception. *Pain*, 2013, 154(1):124-134.

Lee, M. A. *Smoke Signals: A Social History of Marijuana,* New York: Scribner. 2012.

Limebeer, C.L., and Parker, L.A. Delta-9-tetrahydrocannabinol interferes with the establishment and the expression of conditioned rejection reactions produced by cyclophosphamide: a rat model of nausea. *Neuroreport,* (1999, December 16) 10(19), 3769-72.

Lucas, P. Cannabis as an adjunct to or substitute for opiates in the treatment of chronic pain. *Journal of Psychoactive Drugs,* 44(2), April-June, 2012, 125-33.

Machado Rocha, F.C., Stefano, S.C., De Cassia Haiek, R., Rosa Oliveira, L.M., and Da Silveira, D.X. (2008, September). Therapeutic use of Cannabis sativa on chemotherapy-induced nausea and vomiting among cancer patients: systematic review and meta-analysis. *European Journal of Cancer Care,* 17(5), 431-43.

McGhee, Paul. *Humor: The Lighter Path to Resilience and Health,* Author House, 2010.

Mechoulam, Raphael, & David Panikashvili, Esther Shoham. Cannabinoids and Brain Injury: Therapeutic Implications, *Trends in Molecular Medicine,* Feb. 2002, Vol. 8, no. 2, pg. 58–61.

Millichap, J. G. Cannabidiol-Enriched Cannabis for Refractory Epilepsy. *AAP Grand Rounds*, 2014, 31(3), 36-36. doi:10.1542/gr.31-3-36.

Miriam Fishbein, & Sahar Gov, Fadi Assaf, Mikhal Gafni, Ora Keren, Yosef Sarne. Long-term behavioral and biochemical effects of an ultra-low dose of Δ9-tetrahydrocannabinol (THC): neuroprotection and ERK signaling. *Experimental Brain Research*, 2012; 221 (4): 437.

Nauck, F., Klaschik, E. (2004, June). Cannabinoids in the treatment of the cachexia-anorexia syndrome in palliative care patients. *Schmerz*, 18(3), 197-202.

Nelson, K., Walsh, D., Deeter, P., and Sheehan, F. (1994). A phase II study of delta-9-tetrahydrocannabinol for appetite stimulation in cancer-associated anorexia. *Journal of Palliative Care*, 10(1), 14-8.

Noyes, R Jr, & SF Brunk, DA Baram, A. Canter. Analgesic effect of delta-9-tetracannabinol. *Journal of Clinical Pharmacology*, 1975, 15:139-143.

Palmer. Nathan. Do You Have to Learn How to Get High?, The Society Pages, *Sociological Images*, July 2014.

Parker, L.A., Rock, E.M., and Limbeer, C.L. (2011, August). Regulation of nausea and vomiting by cannabinoids. British *Journal of Pharmacology*, 163(7), 1411-22.

Pryce, G., & DR Siddall, DL Selwood, G. Giovannoni, D. Baker. Neuroprotection in Experimental Autoimmune Encephalomyelitis and Progressive Multiple Sclerosis by Cannabis-Based Cannabinoids. *J Neuroimmune Pharmacol.* 2015 Jun;10(2):281-92.

Reiter, Russel J., & Jo Robinson. Melatonin and Marijuana, *Your Body's Natural Wonder Drug*, Bantam Books, 1995.

Russo EB. Cannabinoids in the management of difficult to treat pain. *Therapeutics and Clinical Risk Management.* 2008;4(1):245-259.

Scharff, Constance, Marijuana: The Gateway Drug Myth, *Psychology Today*, Aug. 2014.

Segal, B. *Perspectives on Drug use in the United States*. Philadelphia, PA: Haworth Press. 1986.

Seniors are filling their prescriptions—at a pot shop, *CBS-This Morning*, May 2016.

Singh, Archana & Nishi Misra. Loneliness, depression andsociability in old age, *Ind Psychiatry J.*, 2009 Jan-Jun, 18 (1) 51-55.

Ständer, S., & M. Schmelz, D. Metze, T. Luger, R. Rukwied, R. Distribution of cannabinoid receptor 1 (CB1) and 2 (CB2) on sensory nerve fibers and adnexal structures in human skin. *Journal of Dermatological Science*, 38(3), 177-188.

Talise, Jasen. Marijuana As Muse: How Cannabis and Novelty-Seeking Affect Your Health, *Science, Medicine, Health*, Spring 2011.

Venosa, Ali, How Weighted Blanket Therapy Can Help Those With Anxiety, Autism, And More, *Medical Daily*, 2016.

Vitiello, Michael V. Aging and Sleep, *National Sleep Foundation*, Dec 2009.

Wei, D., & D. Lee, CD Cox, CA Karsten, O Peñagarikano, DH Geschwind, D Piomelli. Endocannabinoid signaling mediates oxytocin-driven social reward. Sept. 2015.

Welty, Timothy, & Adrienne Luebke, Barry Gidal. Cannabidiol: Promise and Pitfalls, *American Epilepsy Society*, Sep-Oct, 2014.

Wilsey, B., Marcotte, T., Deutsch, R., Gouaux, B., Sakai, S., and Donaghe, H. (2013, February). Low-dose vaporized cannabis significantly improves neuropathic pain. *The Journal of Pain*, 14(2), 136-48.

Zajicek, J.P. & VI Apostu. Role of cannabinoids in multiple sclerosis. *CNS Drugs*. 2011, Mar: 25 (3), 187-201.

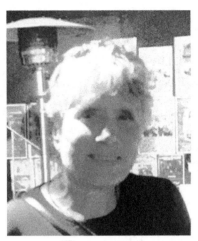

Docpotter

Beverly A. Potter, PhD ("Docpotter") earned her doctorate in counseling psychology from Stanford University and her masters in vocational rehabilitation counseling from San Francisco State University. She is a corporate trainer, public speaker and has authored numerous books on health and workplace issues like overcoming job burnout, managing yourself for excellence, high performance goal setting, mediating conflict, healing magic of cannabis, marijuana recipies (as Mary Jane Stawell), drug testing for employers and passing the test for employees.

Docpotter is based in Oakland, California. Her website—docpotter.com—is packed with useful information. Please visit.

Other Books by Docpotter

The Healing Magic of Cannabis
It's the High that Heals!

Marijuana Recipies & Remedies for Healthy Living
as Mary Jane Stawell

Overcoming Job Burnout:
How To Renew Enthusiasm For Work

Finding A Path With A Heart:
How To Go From Burnout To Bliss

The Worrywart's Companion:
21 Ways to Soothe Yourself & Worry Smart

From Conflict To Cooperation:
How To Mediate A Dispute

Get Peak Performance Every Day:
How to Manage Like a Coach

High Performance Goal Setting:
Using Intuition to Conceive & Achieve Your Dreams

Brain Boosters:
Foods & Drugs That Make You Smarter

Drug Testing At Work:
A Guide For Employers And Employees

Pass the Test: An Employee Guide to Drug Testing

The Way Of The Ronin:
Riding The Waves Of Change At Work

Turning Around:
Keys To Motivation And Productivity

Preventing Job Burnout: A Workbook

Youth Extension A-Z

Beyond Consciousness:
What Happens After Death

Patriots Handbook

Spiritual Secrets for Playing the Game of Life

Simple Pleasures

Question Authority to Think for Yourself

Managing Yourself for Excellence
How to Become a Can-Do Person

Healing Hormones